T0211485

COMMON LIVER DISEASES AND TRANSPLANTATION

An Algorithmic Approach to Work-Up and Management

COMMON LIVER DISEASES AND TRANSPLANTATION

An Algorithmic Approach to Work-Up and Management

EDITED BY

Robert S. Brown Jr, MD, MPH
Frank Cardile Professor of Medicine
Chief, Center for Liver Disease and Transplantation
Columbia University College of Physicians and Surgeons
New York-Presbyterian Hospital
New York, NY

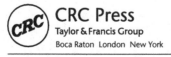
CRC Press
Taylor & Francis Group
Boca Raton London New York

CRC Press is an imprint of the
Taylor & Francis Group, an **informa** business

First published in 2013 by SLACK Incorporated

Published 2024 by CRC Press
2385 NW Executive Center Drive, Suite 320, Boca Raton FL 33431

and by CRC Press
4 Park Square, Milton Park, Abingdon, Oxon, OX14 4RN

CRC Press is an imprint of Taylor & Francis Group, LLC

Library of Congress Cataloging-in-Publication Data

Common liver disease and transplantation : an algorithmic approach to work-up and management / [edited by] Robert S. Brown Jr.
   p. ; cm.
  Includes bibliographical references and index.
  ISBN 978-1-55642-903-3 (alk. paper)
  I. Brown, Robert S., 1963-
  [DNLM: 1. Liver Diseases--diagnosis. 2. Liver Diseases--therapy. 3. Liver Neoplasms. 4. Liver Transplantation. WI 700]

  616.3'62--dc23

          2012040214

ISBN: 9781556429033 (pbk)
ISBN: 9781003523239 (ebk)

DOI: 10.1201/9781003523239

DEDICATION

I would like to dedicate this book to my former students, residents, and fellows who inspired me to write a book that reflected my clinical approach to most liver problems. I hope I have taught you as much as you have taught me.

CONTENTS

ACKNOWLEDGMENTS

Many people need to be acknowledged for the production of this book. First, I am thankful to my coauthors, collaborators, and readers who have produced this material. I think you have made it possible to produce a top-rate educational product that will provide a lasting impact on the readers and future generations of physicians and gastroenterologists/hepatologists. I could not have produced this book without you.

Second, I would like to acknowledge my mentors and teachers and those who have taught me a careful way of approaching medical problems. Particularly, I would like to highlight my mentors in transplantation, Jack Lake, Nancy Ascher, John Roberts, and Jean Emond, who have been friends and collaborators since my early days as a hepatologist.

I would also like to thank Dr. Sanjiv Chopra, who graciously provided the Foreword for this book and is the first person to teach me about liver disease in a careful, algorithmic way. I remember his A through E algorithms for many liver diseases to this day. I enjoy every interaction I have with him. He and many other physicians at the Beth Israel Hospital in Boston instilled a love for gastroenterology and hepatology that has and continues to evolve.

Finally, my finest teacher in medicine has always been my father, Dr. Robert Brown. Not only has he taught me the most about being a physician, but also the importance and reward of teaching younger physicians how to think about medicine in a critical manner. I would also like to thank my mother, without whom I probably would have never finished high school nevermind college or medical school. Your encouragement, cajoling, and support were always invaluable.

I would like to thank my partners here at the Center for Liver Disease and Transplantation at New York-Presbyterian Hospital who have worked with me for the past 14 years and helped build what I think is one of the finest liver programs in the country. I am proud to call you colleagues and friends and thank you for all your support, including tolerating all of the time I spent doing outside ventures.

I would like to thank my publishers at SLACK Incorporated, Carrie Kotlar in particular, without whose ongoing advocacy and support this book would probably never have come to fruition.

I would also like to thank all of the fellows, residents, and students I have had the opportunity to teach over the last 2 decades. Being able to bask in your reflected glory and watching your academic progress and accomplishments is my greatest professional accomplishment. I hope I have been as inspiring to you as you have been to me.

Lastly and most importantly, I would like to thank my family: my children, Jake, Dylan, Jacqueline, and Peyton, and my lovely wife, Sarah. Though my love for you makes it hard to leave each day to go to work, it also inspires me to try to do great things.

ABOUT THE EDITOR

Robert S. Brown Jr, MD, MPH, is the Frank Cardile Professor of Medicine at Columbia University's College of Physicians and Surgeons and the Chief of the Center for Liver Disease and Transplantation at New York-Presbyterian Hospital. He was a co-founder of the Liver Center, a joint program between Weill Cornell and Columbia University, which has grown into the largest liver transplant program in the region and one of the top 5 in the United States. He received his bachelor's degree from Harvard College in Cambridge, Massachusetts, his medical degree from New York University in New York City, and his master's degree in public health from the Graduate School of Public Health at the University of California Berkeley. He completed his internship and residency at Harvard's Beth Israel Hospital in Boston, and Gastroenterology and Hepatology Fellowship at the University of California San Francisco.

Dr. Brown is an active researcher, teacher, and clinician. He has published extensively in liver disease and transplantation, with over 125 peer-reviewed manuscripts and 60 reviews and book chapters. He has edited several books and is an associate editor for the journal *Liver Transplantation*. He is an internationally known teacher and speaker with frequent invited lectures at national and international meetings on liver disease topics. He received the prestigious Senior Attending Teaching Award at Columbia University and many of his former trainees now lead liver transplant programs in the United States and abroad. He served as chair of the national committee to develop guidelines for living donor liver transplantation for the United Network for Organ Sharing. He has a very active clinical practice dedicated to liver disease patients, has been selected as the American Liver Foundation Physician of the Year, and has been one of *New York Magazine's* Top Doctors every year since 2009. He lives in New York with his wife, Sarah, his children, Jacqueline, Peyton, Dylan, and Jake, along with 2 dogs, a cat, and a variable number of fish.

Contributing Authors

George G. Abdelsayed, MD, FACP, FACG (Chapter 1)
Associate Clinical Professor of Medicine
Yale University School of Medicine
Chief and Program Director
Section of Gastroenterology
Bridgeport Hospital
Bridgeport, Connecticut

Patrick Basu, MD, MRCP, AGAF (Chapters 9, 10)
Assistant Professor of Medicine
Columbia University College of Physicians and Surgeons
New York-Presbyterian Hospital
New York, New York

Blaire E. Burman, MD (Chapter 6)
Gastroenterology Research Fellow
University of California San Francisco
Department of Gastroenterology and Hepatology
San Francisco, California

Sanjiv Chopra, MBBS, MACP (Foreword)
Professor of Medicine
Faculty Dean for Continuing Education
Harvard Medical School
Senior Consultant in Hepatology
Beth Israel Deaconess Medical Center
Boston, Massachusetts

Michael Einstein, MD (Chapter 1)
Department of Hepatology and Gastroenterology
Hartford Hospital
Hartford, Connecticut

Scott A. Fink, MD, MPH, FACP (Chapter 8)
Chief, Section of Hepatology
Division of Gastroenterology
Department of Medicine
Main Line Health System
Lankenau Medical Center
Wynnewood, Pennsylvania

Mark W. Russo, MD, MPH, FACG, AGAF (Chapters 3, 4)
Clinical Professor of Medicine
Chief, Division of Hepatology
Medical Director of Liver Transplantation
Carolinas Medical Center
Charlotte, North Carolina

Niraj James Shah, MD (Chapters 9, 10)
Research Assitant
Hofstra Medical School
Department of Medicine
Forest Hills Hospital
New York, New York

Eva Urtasun Sotil, MD (Chapter 2)
Assistant Professor of Clinical Medicine
Medical Director, Living Donor Liver Transplant Program
Columbia University College of Physicians and Surgeons
New York-Presbyterian Hospital
New York, New York

James F. Trotter, MD (Chapter 5)
Baylor University Medical Center
Dallas, Texas

Elizabeth C. Verna, MD, MS (Chapter 7)
Assistant Professor of Medicine
Center for Liver Disease and Transplantation
Division of Digestive and Liver Diseases
Columbia University College of Physicians and Surgeons
New York-Presbyterian Hospital
New York, New York

FOREWORD

I have spent my entire clinical career caring for patients with liver disease and teaching students and trainees about how to best approach the work-up and treatment of liver problems. Despite the large number of textbooks dedicated to liver disease, there is a need for a simple, comprehensive manual of how to adroitly and efficiently care for common liver problems. When Dr. Robert Brown Jr, one of my former trainees, told me that he had not only written such a book but that he wanted me to write the foreword, I was honored that I had played a part in providing inspiration for him to write the book and that he wanted me to be his first reader. I was not disappointed. This book emulates what I have always taught about liver disease. Each chapter in this book has a simple algorithm that allows physicians to quickly and cost-effectively approach common liver problems, get to the right diagnosis, and then provide the appropriate treatment.

Dr. Brown and his coauthors provide a succinct, easy-to-understand approach to most liver diseases, including liver transplant candidates and recipients. Readers, including gastroenterologists, primary care providers, and trainees interested in liver disease, will find the text enormously instructive. It provides a quick how-to guide for anyone who is faced with a liver problem, whether simple or complex. I found the book easy to read and yet detailed enough to provide useful information to virtually any level of practitioner. This book should be on the shelf of every gastroenterologist, GI fellow, and primary care doctor interested in providing the most effective care to their liver patients. Though it provides a simple "cookbook" style, the information is no way simplistic. Pathophysiology, the most recent treatment data, and all clinical care algorithms and societal recommendations are summarized in a comprehensive way.

We all have our textbooks, online resources, and other ways we choose to get clinical information. *Common Liver Diseases and Transplantation* will be the way many of us will choose to learn and adopt new algorithms in liver disease. I suspect Dr. Brown's algorithms will be used for teaching many physicians. I am proud of so many of my prior students and trainees. One of the greatest pleasures we have as teachers is to see our trainees go on to great careers and train others; I am proud to count Dr. Brown among them.

Sanjiv Chopra, MBBS, MACP
Professor of Medicine
Faculty Dean for Continuing Education
Harvard Medical School
Senior Consultant in Hepatology
Beth Israel Deaconess Medical Center
Boston, Massachusetts

INTRODUCTION

This book is intended primarily for practicing gastroenterologists and internists to provide a broad but comprehensive introduction and approach to common liver diseases. It would also be useful for students and trainees interested in internal medicine, gastroenterology/hepatology, and general surgery at virtually every level. I have hoped that the book will provide a review that is comprehensive enough to provide the intellectual basis for the data, yet simple enough to allow people to read it rapidly and assimilate its approach to common liver problems into their clinical practice. Each chapter is intended to be useful and functional as a stand-alone as well as part of an overall picture of approach to liver disease and liver management. As a result, there may be some redundancy between chapters as the approach to many liver diseases is overlapping. I hope you will forgive any redundancy as it was necessary in order to have each chapter be complete, and certainly learning occurs better when important themes are repeated. There is an intended flow; the early chapters are summaries and helpful to read first as a preface. These themes are repeated, modified, and expanded by the liver disease-specific chapters that follow. Each chapter provides background information as well as tables, algorithms, and simple management approaches. Though it is impossible to cover every circumstance that might arise and no book can serve as a replacement for sound clinical judgment, this book does reflect decades of experience managing thousands of patients with these problems. I hope the material will provide a foundation for the generalist who sees very little liver disease and younger physicians with an interest in gastroenterology and hepatology, and hone the experience and update gastroenterologists and surgeons who see liver disease in their practice. I welcome any suggestions that we can incorporate into future editions and once again hope that you learn as much reading it as I did writing and editing it.

PREFACE

I began teaching clinical liver disease in 1995 across 3 institutions spanning the United States. In these 17 years, I have spent innumerable hours teaching in formal and informal formats about common problems in liver disease. Much of this time was spent on rounds or informal "chalk talks" with the residents and fellows. I have always tried to approach clinical problems in a simple, algorithmic way. My informal lectures always included many barely legible diagrams I would write on the chalkboard (now a white board that rarely has a good eraser!) showing how I thought about and approached clinical problems and the common decision points. This strategy was built on the foundation of my mentors. From early on, I was influenced by my father, one of the most thoughtful and careful clinical nephrologists. He taught generations of trainees who to this day remark on his ability to teach about clinical problems. Other mentors at the Beth Israel Hospital in Boston and the University of California San Francisco have helped clarify and modify my approach and taught me about hepatology and transplantation.

When I was asked to write a book summarizing almost 2 decades of teaching how to think about clinical liver problems, I chose my former students and mentees to help me write it. I wanted the book to reflect not my approach to common liver problems, but *our* approach to common liver problems. It is through educating our students and trainees that we, as professors and mentors, learn and refine how we think about problems; this changes as we teach them over time. As a result, the goal of this book is not to present *the* way to *deal* with clinical liver problems, but a way to *think* about clinical liver problems. Please use the material within this book as a foundation for your approach to liver disease that will evolve over time and change with new data, new literature, and your experience with particular patient populations.

I am sure over the next 17 years, I will continue to learn from my patients, my students and trainees, and my colleagues. I hope this book is as useful to you when reading it as it was to me in writing it.

1

Evaluation and Management of Early Liver Disease

Robert S. Brown Jr, MD, MPH; Michael Einstein, MD; and George G. Abdelsayed, MD, FACP, FACG

Liver disease is a common problem in the United States. For example, over 7 million Americans likely have chronic hepatitis B, chronic hepatitis C, or alcoholic liver disease. It is also estimated that nonalcoholic fatty liver disease affects nearly 1 out of 3 people, a prevalence that will continue to increase along with the obesity epidemic. Given that liver disease can lead to cirrhosis, hepatocellular carcinoma, and markedly reduce life expectancy, an appropriate screening algorithm is essential.

Cost-effective and minimally invasive screening tests are essential in today's medical climate. However, diagnosing liver disease can be a challenge especially when the majority of patients present with asymptomatic disease. In its early stages, liver disease is insidious. It silently destroys the liver for months and decades before sequelae become apparent. Identifying liver disease in its early stages and treating it can reduce morbidity and mortality. Similarly, diagnosing viral hepatitis can lead to prevention of spread to others.

WHO AND WHAT TO TEST

Liver disease is common in the population and can be screened for with very simple blood and radiologic testing. Given that liver disease is a major cause of morbidity and mortality, particularly in patients between the ages of

Brown RS Jr. *Common Liver Diseases and Transplantation:*
An Algorithmic Approach to Work-Up and Management (pp 1-15).
© 2013 Taylor & Francis Group.

45 and 65, knowledge of the risk factors for chronic liver disease and an appropriate screening algorithm is essential. As part of their routine general medical evaluation, liver enzymes should be tested, including alanine aminotransferase (ALT), aspartate aminotransferase (AST), alkaline phosphatase, total bilirubin, and albumin levels. ALT and AST do not measure liver function but rather are markers of hepatocyte dysfunction and death. ALT is more specific for liver disease while AST can be elevated in a variety of non-hepatic-related disorders, particularly necrosis of skeletal muscle and hemolysis.

Alkaline phosphatase can be elevated in biliary ductal and infiltrative disorders as well as other nonhepatic diseases. To differentiate hepatic from nonhepatic etiologies the concentration of alkaline phosphatase isoenzymes or level of gamma-glutamyltransferase (GGT), which is liver specific, can be measured. Though GGT is quite specific for liver disease, an important caveat is that many medications as well as alcohol use or minimal hepatic steatosis can induce GGT, thus decreasing its specificity for significant liver disease. Therefore, GGT should not be used routinely to screen for liver disease.

The sensitivity and specificity of these tests depends on the cutoff used. It has been proposed that for monitoring and treating patients with hepatitis B an ALT of 19 IU/mL for women and 30 IU/mL for men be used instead of the "normal" lab cutoffs, which vary from lab to lab.[1] ALT varies by gender, body mass index (BMI), and measures of glucose intolerance. The upper limits of normal in most labs tend to be higher as they are standardized from the general population, which invariably has a proportion of patients with non-alcoholic fatty liver disease. Many experts have adopted these lower values as the general cutoff for screening for liver disease. Those with even mild elevation in aminotransferases do need at least a basic work-up for liver disease.

As some patients with liver disease will have normal liver biochemistries, it is important to be able to identify high-risk populations and use additional screening techniques. A patient's history should be reviewed for risk factors that may predispose him or her to liver disease (Table 1-1). This includes taking a good social history for parenteral drug use and sexual exposures for viral hepatitis risks as well as alcohol use. A detailed review of all prescription medications, over-the-counter medications, vitamins, supplements, and herbal preparations is needed to exclude hepatotoxic exposures. A careful family history is needed for potential genetic liver disorders, including both hepatic and nonhepatic diseases (eg, chronic obstructive pulmonary disease [COPD] in nonsmoking family members would suggest a diagnosis of alpha-1-antitrypsin deficiency). More specific serologic testing should be initiated if risk factors are identified, independent of liver function test (LFT) abnormalities, and these are described in subsequent chapters.

Table 1-1

Risk Factors

MEDICAL HISTORY	ASSOCIATED LIVER DISEASE
Autoimmune diseases (eg, lupus)	Autoimmune hepatitis
History of blood transfusion	HBV, HCV
Dialysis	HBV, HCV
Hypertension, DM, hyperlipidemia	NAFLD
COPD	Alpha-1-antitrypsin
Sarcoidosis, amyloidosis	Infiltrative disease
Cancer	Metastatic cancer
Pregnancy	Pregnancy-related liver disorders
SOCIAL HISTORY	
Country of origin or parents' country of origin	HBV (Asia, Africa, Eastern Europe, the Middle East, South Pacific, Arctic, and most countries in South and Central America)
Illicit drugs, especially IV drugs but also marijuana and intranasal cocaine	HBV, HCV
Alcohol	Alcoholic liver disease
Prison	HBV, HCV
Tattoos or body piercings	HBV, HCV
MSM	HBV, HCV
Household contacts with viral hepatitis	HBV
Recent travel	HAV, HEV
FAMILY HISTORY	
Children born to HCV-infected mother	HCV
Children born to HBV-infected mother	HBV
Genetic disorders	Wilson's disease, hemachromatosis
MEDICATIONS	
Prescription	
Methotrexate, phenytoin	
Azathioprine	Hepatic fibrosis

(continued)

Table 1-1 *(continued)*

Risk Factors

MEDICATIONS	ASSOCIATED LIVER DISEASE
Prescription	
Anesthetics, azathioprine, bone marrow transplant regimens	Sinusoidal obstruction syndrome (veno-occlusive disease)
Antibiotics	Cholestasis
Over-the-Counter	
Acetaminophen	Acute liver failure
NSAIDs	
Vitamin A	
Niacin	
Herbal	
Kava-Kava	Acute liver failure
Skullcap	
Jamaican bush tea	

DM, diabetes mellitus; COPD, chronic obstructive pulmonary disease; NAFLD, nonalcoholic fatty liver disease; MSM, men who have sex with men; HCV, hepatitis C virus; HBV, hepatitis B virus; NSAIDs, nonsteroidal anti-inflammatory drugs.

For patients who will begin chemotherapy or an anti-TNF agent for Crohn's disease, ulcerative colitis, or rheumatoid arthritis, hepatitis B serologies should be checked in all individuals even in the absence of abnormal LFTs or clear risk factors. These patients are at a high risk for having a hepatitis flare if they are not placed on prophylactic oral antiviral therapy.

PATTERNS OF LIVER DISEASE

When a patient has abnormal liver tests at presentation, it is helpful to classify the patient's condition as seen in Table 1-2. This can aid in focusing the differential diagnosis and guiding the subsequent work-up. Even a single abnormal ALT reading should prompt evaluation for hepatitis C, hepatitis B, and hemochromatosis given the high prevalence of these diseases (Table 1-3). If the elevation of aminotransferases is <3x ULN, a period of observation may be reasonable if these initial screening tests are negative, with LFTs repeated regularly for 4 to 6 months if the patient has all of the following:

Table 1-2

Key Questions in Evaluating Abnormal Liver Function Tests

1. Is this problem acute or chronic?
2. Is it a hepatitic or cholestatic pattern?
3. Are there any other comorbidities that need to be considered?
4. Is the patient immunosuppressed?

Table 1-3

Tests for All Patients With Suspected Liver Disease or an Elevated Alanine Aminotransferase

- Hepatitis C antibody by enzyme-linked immunosorbent assay (ELISA)
- Hepatitis B surface antigen (HBsAg) and hepatitis B core antibody (anti-HBc)
- Iron, total iron binding capacity, and ferritin for hereditary hemochromatosis

- Preserved synthetic function.
- No identifiable risk factors for liver disease.
- Negative initial screening tests.
- No evidence of biliary obstruction.
- The patient is asymptomatic. During this period, both alcohol and other potential hepatotoxins should be avoided.

ACUTE LIVER INJURY

Acute liver injury occurs over a period of less than 3 to 6 months and encompasses both mild, usually reversible conditions, as well as acute liver failure defined as coagulopathy and encephalopathy in the absence of pre-existing liver disease, which has high mortality without urgent transplantation. These illnesses are typically hallmarked by high levels of AST and

ALT (>1000 U/L) and are frequently symptomatic (abdominal pain, fatigue, nausea, jaundice, anorexia).

Disorders that typically cause this degree of liver inflammation are acute viral hepatitis (hepatitis A, B, D, E; rarely C), Wilson's disease, ischemia or "shock liver," autoimmune hepatitis, drug-induced liver injury, pregnancy-associated liver disease (hemolysis, elevated liver enzymes, and low platelets [HELLP]; acute fatty liver of pregnancy; cholestasis of pregnancy), and Budd-Chiari syndrome. Alcoholic hepatitis will not have an ALT above 500 and typically has an AST:ALT ratio of >2. A transient increase in ALT can also result from a passing gallstone through the common bile duct.

Aminotransferase levels significantly higher than 5000 U/L usually are due to acetaminophen hepatotoxicity, ischemic hepatitis, or viral hepatitis such as from herpesvirus. For aminotransferases around 1000, the differential diagnosis includes acute viral hepatitis, Wilson's disease, shock liver, autoimmune hepatitis, alcoholic hepatitis, drug/toxin-induced liver injury, pregnancy-associated liver diseases, and Budd-Chiari syndrome. Figure 1-1 outlines an algorithm for hepatitis work-up. The specific tests to order for acute liver injury are shown in Table 1-4 and should also include a Doppler ultrasound of the liver to assess the hepatic vessels.

CHRONIC LIVER INJURY

Categorizing chronic liver injury into hepatitic versus cholestatic, as well as examining the degree of elevation can aid in directing the work-up. Knowing the chronicity and degree of aminotransferase elevation will further focus the differential and evaluation. The additional tests to order based on clinical suspicion are shown in Table 1-5.

Chronic Hepatitic Liver Disease

The majority of chronic liver diseases are hepatitic in nature. The most common diagnoses are viral hepatitis B (HBV) and viral hepatitis C (HCV), alcoholic and nonalcoholic fatty liver diseases, hemochromatosis, and autoimmune liver disease. Less common diseases include hepatitis D (which occurs only in patients with HBV), alpha-1-antitrypsin deficiency, and Wilson's disease. These tend to be hepatitis and are marked by aminotransferase (AST, ALT) elevation more than alkaline phosphatase. Most mild elevations in LFTs (2 to 10x ULN) are found incidentally on screening. With the exception of alcoholic liver disease, the ALT will be greater than the AST except when advanced fibrosis or cirrhosis is present. Without an identifiable risk factor and continued elevation of LFTs

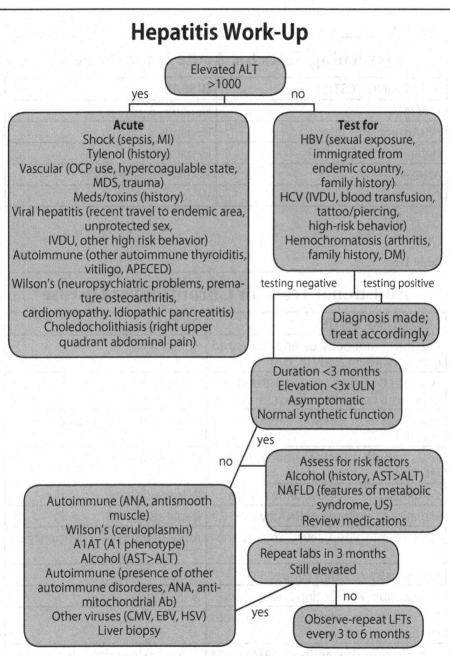

Figure 1-1. Algorithm for initial work-up of hepatitis.

Table 1-4

Screening Tests for Acute Liver Disease

SCREENING TEST(S)	DISEASE
HAV IgM	Hepatitis A
HBsAg, anti-HBc IgM	Hepatitis B
Hepatitis C RNA by PCR	Hepatitis C
ANA, anti-LKM	Autoimmune hepatitis
Ceruloplasmin, serum copper	Wilson's disease

Table 1-5

Additional Tests for Chronic Liver Disease

SCREENING TEST(S)	DISEASE
Hepatitis C antibody by enzyme-linked immunosorbent assay (ELISA)	Hepatitis C
Hepatitis B surface antigen (HBsAg) and hepatitis B core antibody (anti-HBc)	Hepatitis B
Iron, total iron binding capacity, and ferritin	Hereditary hemochromatosis
ANA, smooth muscle antibody (ASMA), IgG level	Autoimmune hepatitis
Ceruloplasmin, 24-hour urine copper	Wilson's disease
Hepatitis D antibody or RNA by PCR	Hepatitis D
Alpha-1-antitrypsin level and phenotype	Alpha-1-antitrypsin deficiency
Ceruloplasmin, serum copper	Wilson's disease
Hemoglobin A1C, fasting lipids	NAFLD
Fasting insulin and glucose, thyroid stimulating hormone	
Antimitochondrial antibody (AMA), IgM level	Primary biliary cirrhosis
pANCA	Primary sclerosing cholangitis
ACE level, chest CT	Sarcoidosis

for over 6 months, further work-up is warranted. Although patients may be asymptomatic, they occasionally complain of fatigue and right upper quadrant pain. The work-up is described in Figure 1-1 and additional testing in Table 1-5.

Chronic Cholestastic Liver Disease

Diseases that primarily affect the biliary system are termed *cholestatic diseases*. The primary biochemical abnormality is alkaline phosphatase elevation. This is due to a reactive proliferation of bile ducts and synthesis of alkaline phosphatase from hepatocytes, rather than necrosis and release of enzymes from damaged cells. Diseases can affect the small intrahepatic ducts, the larger extrahepatic ducts, or both. Typically middle-aged females will have primary biliary cirrhosis and those with inflammatory bowel disease will have primary sclerosing cholangitis. Alkaline phosphatase can also be elevated due to infiltrative disorders such as sarcoidosis, amyloidosis, and lymphoma. Bilirubin can be elevated but can also be elevated with severe hepatocellular disorders like cirrhosis or acute hepatitis. Figure 1-2 outlines the work-up for an elevated alkaline phosphatase or cholestatic liver process and specific tests are in Table 1-5.

PREDICTING DEGREE OF FIBROSIS

Cirrhosis is the end stage of many forms of chronic liver disease and is the 12th leading cause of death in the United States.[2] Prevention of disease progression before cirrhosis is established is the most important task of the physician and patient. Establishing if the patient has cirrhosis during the initial evaluation of all patients with chronic liver disease is essential since subsequent care and management is determined by the initial stage of liver disease. In addition to preventing further progression, it is important to identify and attempt to modify other comorbidities the patient may have. The gold standard to establish the stage of liver disease remains liver biopsy. This may be done percutaneously, transjugularly, or laparoscopically. The most commonly used staging system is the METAVIR system, which assigns a grade (0 to 4 for inflammation) and stage (0 to 4 for fibrosis).[3] The Ishak scoring system grades inflammation from 0 to 4 and fibrosis from 0 to 6 and is commonly used in research studies.[4] For the purpose of this discussion, early liver disease is defined as a stage 0 to 2 on liver biopsy. Although safe, liver biopsy is an invasive procedure and carries some risks, most notably bleeding, which may be fatal in 1 out of 10,000 cases.[5] Therefore, alternatives to liver biopsy have been studied. These noninvasive alternatives are divided into cross-sectional imaging studies and direct and indirect tests (Table 1-6). None are

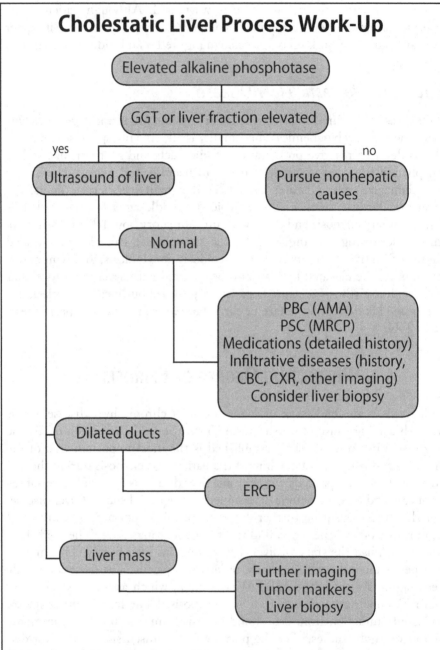

Cholestatic Liver Process Work-Up

Elevated alkaline phosphotase

GGT or liver fraction elevated

yes   no

Ultrasound of liver   Pursue nonhepatic causes

Normal

PBC (AMA)
PSC (MRCP)
Medications (detailed history)
Infiltrative diseases (history,
CBC, CXR, other imaging)
Consider liver biopsy

Dilated ducts

ERCP

Liver mass

Further imaging
Tumor markers
Liver biopsy

GGT, gamma glutamyltransferase; PBC, primary biliary cirrhosis; AMA, antimito-chondrial antibody; PSC, primary sclerosing cholangitis; MRCP, magnetic resonance cholangiopancreatography; CBC, complete blood count; CXR, chest x-ray; ERCP, endoscopic retrograde cholangiopancreatography.

Figure 1-2. Algorithm for work-up of a cholestatic liver process or an elevated alkaline phosphatase.

Table 1-6

Noninvasive Markers of Hepatic Fibrosis/Cirrhosis

SERUM BIOMARKERS		
Indirect	*Direct*	*Cross-Sectional Imaging*
AST	Laminin	CT
ALT	Type I/IV collagens	MRI
APRI (AST/Platelet Ratio Index)	Hyaluronic acid	Ultrasound
FIB-4 index	Matrix metalloproteinases	TE
FibroTest		TE, MRI
FibroSure		

AST, aspartate aminotransferase; ALT, aminotransferase; CT, computed tomography; TE, transient elastography; MRI, magnetic resonance imaging.

currently FDA approved. Indirect tests reflect alterations in hepatic function but do not directly reflect extracellular matrix metabolism. Direct markers of fibrosis reflect extracellular matrix metabolism turnover. Of the cross-sectional imaging tests, the most studied and promising is FibroScan, using the principle of transient elastography (TE). TE is a measure of liver stiffness and is measured in Kilopascals (kPa), utilizing either ultrasound or magnetic resonance imaging (MRI). Further work is underway to standardize these measurements for a variety of conditions, such as hepatitis C and nonalcoholic fatty liver disease (NAFLD). The most common and well-studied disease with FibroScan is hepatitis C, where a cutoff of 7.1 kPa appears to be predictive of significant fibrosis.[6] The main disadvantage of all noninvasive markers of fibrosis is the inability to reliably differentiate early stages from moderate stages of fibrosis.

Basic laboratory values can also be helpful to assess for advanced fibrosis and sometimes may obviate the need for liver biopsy. Many of these methods to estimate the degree of liver fibrosis have been evaluated in a variety of different chronic liver diseases. The specific cutoff for each test depends on the type of liver disease and to what degree of fibrosis is being screened.

Some have advocated the use of an AST/ALT cutoff of >1 to predict cirrhosis. The results of many studies have been inconsistent and in alcoholic liver disease, where the ratio is typically elevated, this model is unreliable.

AST to platelet ratio (APRI) has been studied in many chronic liver disease populations including HCV, HBV, and alcoholic liver disease. In patients with HCV a threshold of 0.7 estimated significant fibrosis with a sensitivity and specificity of 77% and 72%, respectively. When the threshold was increased to 1.0, cirrhosis was predicted with a sensitivity and specificity of 76% and 72%, respectively. In those with HBV a threshold of 0.6 had a sensitivity and specificity of 75.9% and 60.5%, respectively, for predicting cirrhosis. While these methods may not be diagnostic for advanced liver disease, they are inexpensive and can aid in identifying those who are at risk of complications from their liver disease. Thrombocytopenia (using a cutoff of 100 to 150,000) in the absence of hematologic disorders is usually quite specific for advanced fibrosis with portal hypertension leading to splenic sequestration of platelets, but is not sensitive. Splenomegaly on imaging and age, particularly for liver diseases that are vertically transmitted (eg, hepatitis B), also predict advanced disease.

RADIOLOGIC TESTING

Hepatic imaging has a limited but useful role in the evaluation of patients with liver disease. Ultrasound is a fast, inexpensive, noninvasive, radiation-free modality that can help detect a variety of liver disorders. It is an excellent test to look for proximal gallstones (particularly in the gallbladder) with a sensitivity of near 90%. However, distal stones in the common bile duct can be obscured by bowel gas. In a meta-analysis of predictive factors for choledocholithiasis, ultrasound had a sensitivity of 38% for detecting a common bile duct stone and 42% for detecting biliary dilation. The addition of Doppler interrogation of the hepatic vessels can identify vascular abnormalities like Budd-Chiari syndrome or portal vein thrombosis. Fatty liver is recognized by ultrasound in the majority of cases with a positive predictive value of 96% and a negative predictive value of 19%.

The sensitivity of ultrasound for detecting metastatic lesions in the liver is poor (53% to 77%), with even lower sensitivity (20%) for lesions <1 cm. For these small lesions, a triple phase computed tomography (CT) with intravenous contrast or a gadolinium contrast enhanced MRI is more sensitive. Other limitations of ultrasound include difficulty assessing morbidly obese patients, patients with respiratory compromise, and patients with steatosis or cirrhosis, as artifact may decrease the sensitivity for some lesions. Despite these limitations, ultrasound should serve as the initial radiologic test to evaluate for liver disease. Triple phase CT with intravenous contrast or gadolinium enhanced MRI should be used to assess any lesions seen on ultrasound screening or when the suspicion of a primary or secondary hepatic malignancy is high.

Magnetic resonance cholangiopancreatography (MRCP) has become the initial screening test of choice in most situations for the presence of biliary tract disease and has largely replaced diagnostic endoscopic retrograde cholangiopancreatography (ERCP). ERCP should be reserved for instances where the pretest probability of a common bile duct stone, biliary obstruction, or stricturing disease requiring intervention is high. Percutaneous transhepatic cholangiography is used instead of ERCP in patients with altered intestinal anatomy (Roux-en-Y choledochojejunostomy) or when lesions above the liver hilum not amenable to endoscopic therapy are found.

GENERAL CARE OF THE PATIENT WITH LIVER DISEASE

All patients with chronic liver disease and especially those with hepatitis C should be vaccinated against hepatitis A and B if they are not immune (Figure 1-3). Thus, as part of the initial work-up of all patients with chronic hepatitis B, the hepatitis A total antibody (not IgM for acute HAV) should be obtained to assess for the presence of immunity. Asymptomatic immunity rises with age up to 60% in some patients. Furthermore, in patients without HBV, screening for hepatitis B core total antibody (anti-HBc) and hepatitis B surface antibody (anti-HBs) to look for either natural immunity (anti-HBc positive with or without anti-HBs) or vaccination-induced immunity (anti-HBc negative, anti-HBs positive) is indicated. Once again total anti-HBc must be determined as anti-HBc IgM will be negative with prior HBV infection. Patients should be vaccinated with the appropriate monoviral (HAV or HBV) vaccine or combination hepatitis A/B vaccine. It is also recommended that patients with early liver disease receive the influenza vaccine on an annual basis and Pneumovax (Merck, Whitehouse Station, NJ) every 5 years.

The use of medications is often feared and patients with early liver disease should be reassured that they could use almost all medications safely. Much of this fear stems from warning labels on packaging and the media. Two particular agents that need to be addressed are acetaminophen and statins. It is important to know that acetaminophen in therapeutic doses is not toxic to the liver. However, patients who chronically use alcohol or barbiturates, which induces the cytochrome p450 system, may be more sensitive to acetaminophen toxicity and can develop toxicity at lower levels. For patients who are not chronically using alcohol, 500 mg every 4 to 6 hours or up to 2000 mg/day can be safe.[7] For those who are chronically using alcohol, doses as low as 2 to 3 g per day have been shown to be toxic and acetaminophen should be avoided in this group. This is particularly an issue in patients who use combination analgesics with acetaminophen plus narcotics.

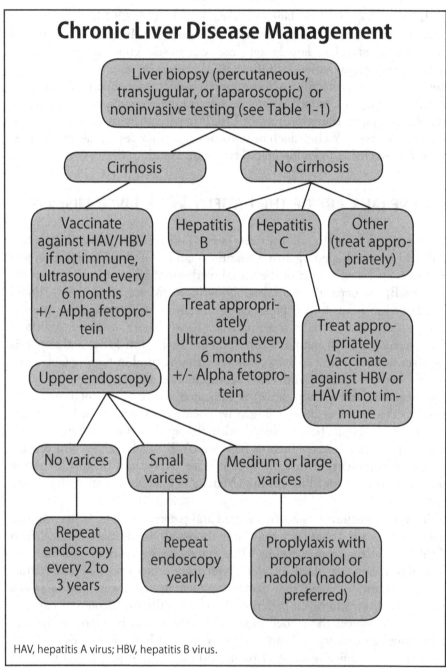

Figure 1-3. Algorithm for management of the chronic liver disease/cirrhotic patient.

Statins can also be used safely in patients with liver disease. The incidence of hepatotoxicity from the statins (and other medications) is generally not higher in patients with liver disease, though the severity may be higher in patients who develop early hepatotoxicity compared to those without liver disease. Many hepatologists will monitor LFTs regularly when initiating statins though the data supporting this practice are absent. For other drugs with significant hepatotoxicity, close monitoring is important. This would be particularly true with drugs such as isoniazid (INH) or methotrexate, which can have an insidious hepatotoxicity.

It is important to caution patients with chronic liver disease against cofactors that will make their liver disease advance more quickly. The most common of these would be alcohol use. It is unclear whether there is a safe alcohol level for patients who have chronic liver disease. It has been shown that binge drinking (ie, more than 3 drinks in 1 session) can lead to fatty deposition in the liver and this has been shown to advance fibrosis progression for hepatitis B and C. Most hepatologists advise alcohol abstinence or a limit of 8 g (1 alcoholic drink) per day.

It is likely also true that nonalcoholic fatty liver disease due to obesity and/or diabetes can also hasten the progression of other liver diseases. In these patients, weight loss, diabetic control, and lipid control should be an issue.

REFERENCES

1. Keeffe EB, Dieterich DT, Han SH, et al. A treatment algorithm for the management of chronic hepatitis B virus infection in the United States: 2008 update. *Clin Gastroenterol Hepatol.* 2008;6(12):1315-1341; quiz 1286.
2. D'Amico G, Garcia-Tsao G, Pagliaro L. Natural history and prognostic indicators of survival in cirrhosis: a systematic review of 118 studies. *J Hepatol.* 2006;44(1):217-231.
3. Bedossa P, Poynard T. An algorithm for the grading of activity in chronic hepatitis C. The METAVIR Cooperative Study Group. *Hepatology.* 1996;24(2):289-293.
4. Ishak KG. Chronic hepatitis: morphology and nomenclature. *Mod Pathol.* 1994;7(6):690-713.
5. Bravo AA, Sheth SG, Chopra S. Liver biopsy. *N Engl J Med.* 2001;344(7):495-500.
6. Castera L. Transient elastography and other noninvasive tests to assess hepatic fibrosis in patients with viral hepatitis. *J Viral Hepat.* 2009;16(5):300-314.
7. Chandok N, Watt KD. Pain management in the cirrhotic patient: the clinical challenge. *Mayo Clin Proc.* 2010;85(5):451-458.

2

Medical Care and Special Considerations for Patients With Advanced Liver Disease/Cirrhosis

Eva Urtasun Sotil, MD

DEFINITION, EPIDEMIOLOGY, CAUSES, NATURAL HISTORY, AND PROGNOSIS

Cirrhosis is defined as the presence of anatomic distortion of the liver parenchyma due to fibrosis deposition with formation of regenerative nodules. It is the final stage of many liver conditions in which persistent inflammation affects the liver parenchyma.

The exact prevalence of cirrhosis in the United States is unknown. The National Institute of Diabetes and Digestive and Kidney Diseases (NIDDK) data estimated the prevalence at 0.15% for the years 1976 to 1980.[1] This number is thought to underrepresent the true prevalence of cirrhosis. It is the 12th leading cause of death in the United States according to the latest National Vital Statistics data.[2]

The most frequent conditions that lead to cirrhosis in the United States are viral hepatitis (hepatitis B and C), alcoholic liver disease, nonalcoholic steatohepatitis, autoimmune hepatitis, and biliary disorders (primary biliary cirrhosis, primary sclerosing cholangitis).

The time frame necessary to develop cirrhosis is extremely variable and depends on the underlying disease and host factors. For hepatitis C, it is

Table 2-1

Child-Turcotte-Pugh Classification

	1 POINT	2 POINTS	3 POINTS
Total bilirubin (mg/dL)*	<2	2 to 3	>3
Albumin (g/dL)	>3.5	2.8 to 3.5	<2.8
PT-INR	<1.7	1.7 to 2.3	>2.3
Ascites	None	Mild	Moderate
Hepatic encephalopathy	None	Grade I to II	Grade III to IV

Child-Turcotte-Pugh class A, 5 to 6 points; class B, 7 to 9; class C, 10 to 15.

For patients with biliary disease (eg, primary biliary cirrhosis or primary sclerosing cholangitis) bilirubin levels: 1 point <4 mg/dL, 2 points 4 to 10 mg/dL, and 3 points >10 mg/dL.

estimated that 5% to 25% will develop cirrhosis over a period of 25 to 30 years of disease.[3] A much faster course is seen with other conditions such as untreated autoimmune hepatitis.

During the first stage of cirrhosis, termed *compensated cirrhosis*, the patient experiences minimal signs and symptoms and may not be aware of the diagnosis. This stage will typically last several years. Eventually portal hypertension and liver synthetic dysfunction worsen and the patient will start to experience signs and symptoms of the disease. Once the patient develops one of the major complications of cirrhosis such as hepatic encephalopathy, variceal bleeding, or ascites, he or she is considered to have progressed to decompensated cirrhosis and survival is significantly shortened from a median of 8.9 years to 1.6 years.[4]

Estimating survival in patients with cirrhosis is critical in determining timing of referral to the only known cure: liver transplantation. Survival can also be assessed using Child-Turcotte-Pugh classification[5] (Table 2-1) and the Model for End-Stage Liver Disease (MELD) (MELD = 3.78 [Ln serum bilirubin {mg/dL}] + 11.2 [Ln INR] + 9.57 [Ln serum creatinine {mg/dL}] + 6.43).[6] The MELD score was first developed as a predictor of 3-month survival in cirrhotic patients following transjugular intrahepatic portosystemic shunt (TIPS), but has been generalized to virtually all forms of liver failure. It has the advantage of being an objective and numeric point system, extensively validated in the literature and the current system used by the United Network for Organ Sharing (UNOS) to prioritize patients for organ allocation.

WHEN TO REFER FOR LIVER TRANSPLANT EVALUATION

Liver transplantation is a surgical operation in which either a section of or an entire liver is removed from a donor and placed into a recipient in need. It is the only cure for end-stage liver disease/cirrhosis. While liver transplant is the only available cure for established cirrhosis, the morbidity and mortality of the operation and immunosuppression required for organ survival is significant and should be considered before placing a patient on the liver transplant list. The current survival for a cadaveric liver transplant is 85.6% at 1 year and 71.9% at 3 years.[7] Only when the disease's mortality exceeds that of the liver transplant predicted mortality should the patient be listed. This occurs when the patients experience their first episode of decompensation, when they are diagnosed with hepatocellular carcinoma, or when they are above a certain MELD score. Survival benefit is present for MELD scores ≥15, and for MELD scores as low as 12 if high-quality grafts are used.[8,9]

PORTAL HYPERTENSIVE COMPLICATIONS: EVALUATION AND MANAGEMENT

The improvement in survival rates in patients with cirrhosis in the last few decades has been due to the improvements seen in liver transplantation as well as improvements in the management of cirrhosis-related complications. These complications are due to a combination of portal hypertension (HTN) and decreased liver synthetic function. The hyperdynamic circulation seen with progression of portal HTN plays a significant role in most of these complications. Portal HTN leads to arterial splanchnic vasodilatation and decreased peripheral vascular resistance, perceived arterial hypovolemia and activation of the renin-angiotensin-aldosterone system (RAAS), sympathetic nervous system, and excessive production of the antidiuretic hormone.[10] While these systems increase arterial blood volume and tone, they also lead to total body salt and water retention, which in turn worsens portal HTN. Many of the current therapies of the cirrhosis-related complications aim at relieving this intense activation of RAAS and sympathetic nervous system.

This section will describe the current clinical practice based on available guidelines and the author's experience when guidelines are not available or vague.[11-13]

Table 2-2 provides dosing information for the most commonly used medications in patients with cirrhosis.

Table 2-2

Dosing for the Most Commonly Used Medications in Cirrhosis

MEDICATION	INITIAL DOSE	TITRATION
Propranolol	20 mg BID	Titrate to obtain a reduction in resting heart rate of 25% or 55 bpm
Nadolol	40 mg QD	Titrate to obtain a reduction in resting heart rate of 25% or 55 bpm
Carvedilol	6.25 mg QD	Double the dose to 12.5 mg QD in 1 week if systolic blood pressure over 90 mm Hg
Octreotride drip (for bleeding)	50 mcg bolus	Followed by 50 mcg per hour for 5 days
Furosemide	40 mg QD	With spironolactone. Adjust dose based on potassium and creatinine levels
Spirono-lactone	100 mg QD	With furosemide. Adjust dose based on potassium and creatinine levels
Octreotide (for HRS)	100 mcg subcutaneous TID	Double dose to 200 mg subcutaneous TID based on response (rise in blood pressure, reduction in creatinine)
Midodrine (for HRS)	7.5 mg TID	Increase dose to 12.5 mg TID based on response (rise in blood pressure, reduction in creatinine). To be used in combination with octreotide and albumin 25% (20 to 40 g per day)
Tolvaptan	15 mg QD	Double dose every 24 hours to maximum of 60 mg QD if no response (<5 mmol/L increase in serum sodium)
Rifaximin	550 mg BID	No titration
Lactulose	30 cc TID	Titrate to obtain 2 to 3 bowel movements per day
Norfloxacin	400 mg QD	No titration

HRS, hepatorenal syndrome; mg, milligram; cc, cubic centimeter; QD, daily; BID, twice a day; TID, 3 times a day; bpm, beats per minute; mm Hg, millimeters of mercury.

Varices

Varices are enlarged collateral vessels seen anywhere along the gastrointestinal tract. The most common areas in which they form are the esophagus, stomach, and rectum. The highest risk of bleeding is seen for varices in the distal esophagus where the luminal wall is thinnest, followed by the gastric fundus.

When to Screen

Patients with cirrhosis should be screened with an esophagogastroduodenoscopy (EGD) at the time of diagnosis of cirrhosis. If no varices are seen, repeat EGD should be done in 3 years or at the time of decompensation. If small varices are found and no treatment is initiated, the endoscopy is repeated in 1 year. Those patients with decompensated cirrhosis should undergo EGD yearly. The progression of varices from small to medium/large is 7% to 8% per year.

Primary Prophylaxis

If medium or large varices are found, primary prophylaxis for bleeding is recommended. Recommendations on primary prophylaxis for variceal bleeding are described in Figure 2-1. This involves the use of nonselective beta-blockers (propranolol, nadolol, carvedilol) in most cases. Recent data suggests that carvedilol may be more effective than other nonselective beta-blockers in reducing portal HTN and preventing bleeding due to its nonselective beta-blocker and anti-alpha-1 adrenergic properties.[14] In patients with large varices or those that do not tolerate beta blockade, prophylactic endoscopic band ligation can be undertaken. It is important to note that cardioselective beta-blockers should be avoided and nitrates are no longer used for variceal bleeding prophylaxis.

Treatment of Acute Variceal Hemorrhage

Management of an acute variceal hemorrhage is described in Figure 2-2. The management is primarily endoscopic for esophageal variceal bleeding with band ligation. This is usually combined with pharmacologic therapy to reduce portal pressures. An octreotide drip is preferred or vasopressin with a nitrate. For gastric variceal bleeding, the treatment is usually pharmacologic or the placement of a TIPS. Newer endoscopic therapies are being developed for gastric varices including cyanoacrylate injection. TIPS is also indicated for persistent or recurrent variceal bleeding after endoscopic therapy. For all patients with variceal bleeding, prophylactic antibiotics are indicated (a quinolone, third-generation cephalosporin, or piperacillin/tazobactam) to prevent spontaneous bacterial peritonitis (SBP) and other infections. Though correction of coagulopathy and thrombocytopenia is often needed, blood

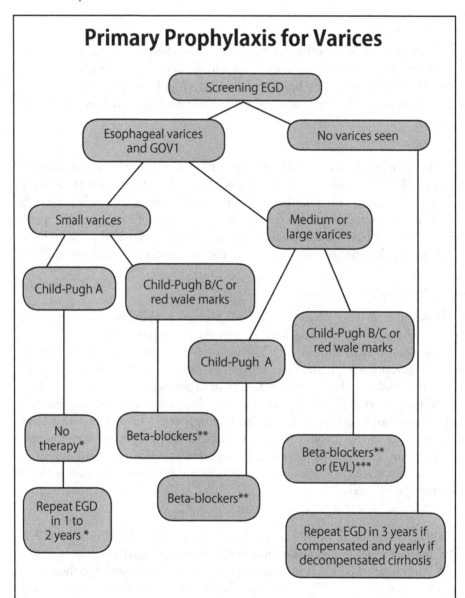

Primary Prophylaxis for Varices

EGD, esophagogastroduodenoscopy; GOV1, gastroesophageal varices category; EVL, endoscopic variceal ligation.

*Beta-blockers are optional in this category as per AASLD guidelines.

**Titrate beta-blockers to HR of 55 to 65 bpm. No further EGD necessary after initiation of beta-blocker therapy. If beta-blockers are not tolerated or contraindicated, EVL can be considered for medium/large esophageal and GOV1 varices.

***For patients undergoing EVL, EGD should be performed every 1 to 2 weeks until eradication of varices, then 1 to 3 months after eradication and every 6 to 12 months thereafter.

Figure 2-1. Primary prophylaxis for varices.

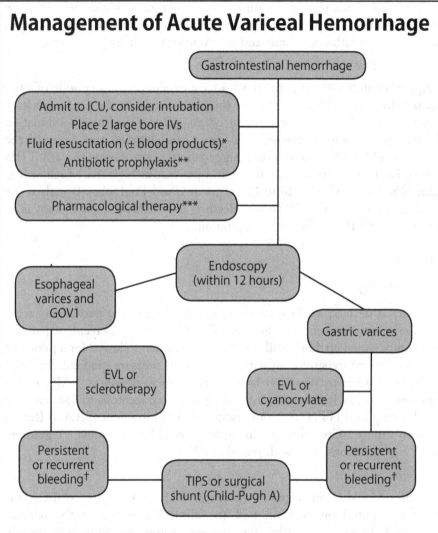

Management of Acute Variceal Hemorrhage

Gastrointestinal hemorrhage

Admit to ICU, consider intubation
Place 2 large bore IVs
Fluid resuscitation (± blood products)*
Antibiotic prophylaxis**

Pharmacological therapy***

Endoscopy
(within 12 hours)

Esophageal
varices and
GOV1

Gastric varices

EVL or
sclerotherapy

EVL or
cyanocrylate

Persistent
or recurrent
bleeding†

TIPS or surgical
shunt (Child-Pugh A)

Persistent
or recurrent
bleeding†

ICU, intensive care unit; IV, intravenous; GOV1, gastroesophageal varices category; EVL, endoscopic variceal ligation; TIPS, transjugular intrahepatic portosystemic shunt.

*Blood products generally given to accomplish INR <1.5, platelet count >50,000/mL and Hgb level 8 to 9 g/dL. rFVIIa generally not used as multicenter placebo-controlled trial showed no benefit.

**Short-term (5 to 7 days) quinolone (oral or IV) use or ceftriaxone in hospitals with high percentage of quinolone-resistant microorganisms.

***Dosages of pharmacotherapeutic agents: somatostatin 50 mcg bolus followed by 50 mcg/hour; terlipressin (not available in US) 2 mg every 4 hours; vasopressin 0.2 to 0.4 units/minute in combination with nitroglycerin 400 μg/minute. Pharmacological therapy should be continued for 3 to 5 days after diagnosis.

†Consider temporary balloon tamponade (not to exceed 24 hours).

Figure 2-2. Management of acute variceal hemorrhage.

products and fluids should be minimized as overresuscitation will increase portal pressures. The need for temporary balloon tamponade is rare in experienced centers with endoscopic and interventional radiologic expertise.

Secondary Prophylaxis

Approximately 50% of patients who have experienced an episode of variceal bleeding will rebleed.[15] Most of the bleeds occur in the first 6 weeks.[16] Secondary prophylaxis is recommended in all cases with a combination of beta-blockers and successive endoscopic band ligation therapy until the varices are obliterated. Recent data suggest better outcomes with early TIPS (within 72 hours) after a variceal bleed in patients at high risk of rebleeding (Child-Pugh class C with 10 to 13 points or Child-Pugh class B with active bleeding at endoscopy).[17] Recurrent bleeding despite endoscopic therapy is an indication for TIPS or liver transplantation.

Ascites

Definition

Ascites is defined as the excess presence of fluid in the peritoneal cavity. It is the most common complication of cirrhosis. Fifty percent of patients with compensated cirrhosis will develop ascites when followed for a period of 10 years.[4] Portal hypertension with hepatic vein pressure gradient (HVPG) levels >10 mm Hg are necessary for the development of ascites.[18] All patients with new onset ascites should have a diagnostic paracentesis to confirm that it is due to portal HTN. A serum ascites albumin gradient (SAAG) (serum albumin minus ascites albumin in mg/dL) should be obtained. A gradient over 1.1 g/dL is consistent with portal HTN.

Management

Ascites should be managed in a stepwise fashion according to the severity of the initial presentation and the clinical response of the patient. Figure 2-3 shows an algorithm for ascites management. Sodium restriction and a combination of a loop diuretic (eg, furosemide) with a potassium-sparing aldosterone-blocking diuretic (eg, spironolactone) are the initial therapies. Patients who do not respond to maximal doses or develop complications of diuretics are managed with TIPS, serial large volume paracentesis, or transplantation. Free water restriction is rarely needed and should be reserved for patients with hyponatremia. Hyponatremia occurs in advanced disease when the amount of water retention is increased compared to the amount of sodium retention due to excessive antidiuretic hormone (ADH) release.[19] This is almost exclusively seen in patients with severe ascites.[20] Hyponatremia can have significant consequences including worsening HE[19] and limits the use of diuretics. Two vasopressor receptor antagonists have been approved for use in

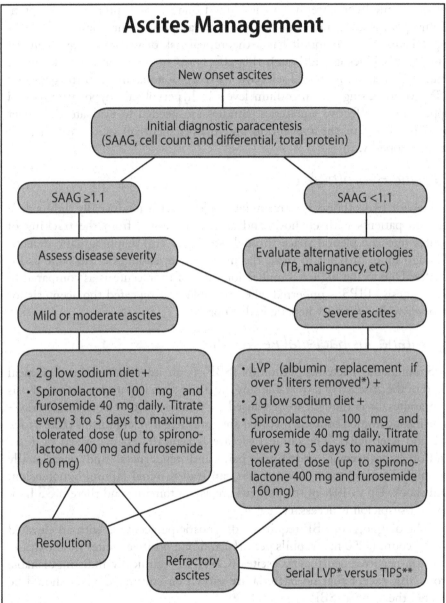

Ascites Management

New onset ascites

Initial diagnostic paracentesis
(SAAG, cell count and differential, total protein)

SAAG ≥1.1

SAAG <1.1

Assess disease severity

Evaluate alternative etiologies
(TB, malignancy, etc)

Mild or moderate ascites

Severe ascites

- 2 g low sodium diet +
- Spironolactone 100 mg and furosemide 40 mg daily. Titrate every 3 to 5 days to maximum tolerated dose (up to spirono-lactone 400 mg and furosemide 160 mg)

- LVP (albumin replacement if over 5 liters removed*) +
- 2 g low sodium diet +
- Spironolactone 100 mg and furosemide 40 mg daily. Titrate every 3 to 5 days to maximum tolerated dose (up to spirono-lactone 400 mg and furosemide 160 mg)

Resolution

Refractory ascites

Serial LVP* versus TIPS**

SAAG, serum ascites albumin gradient; TB, tuberculosis; LVP, large volume paracentesis; TIPS, transjugular intrahepatic portosystemic shunt.

*Removal of over 5 L of fluid via paracentesis can lead to decreased intravascular volume, further activation of RAAS and precipitation of hepatorenal syndrome. Albumin replacement (8g/L of fluid removed) is recommended.

**TIPS can be considered in patients that have no contraindications (no PV thrombosis, good renal, cardiac, and hepatic synthetic function). TIPS results in better control of ascites, more hepatic encephalopathy but has no clear survival benefit.

Figure 2-3. Ascites management.

hypervolemic hyponatremia in the United States, conivaptan and tolvaptan. Conivaptan is an intravenous nonselective vasopressin antagonist. By blocking V1 and V2 receptors it has a theoretical risk of worsening hypotension through V1 blockage, although this effect was not seen on a small clinical study.[21] Tolvaptan is an oral selective V2 receptor antagonist. Both agents are effective in raising serum sodium levels in hypervolemic hyponatremia and appear to be effective aquaretics. Studies are needed to evaluate the effect of these drugs in the prevention and management of ascites and hepatic encephalopathy.

Hepatic Hydrothorax

Hepatic hydrothorax is a transudative pleural effusion (usually right sided) seen in patients with cirrhosis and ascites. It results from the tracking of ascites into the pleural space through small (<1 cm) diaphragmatic defects. Though more difficult to treat, the management should be the same as for ascites. Due to the higher complication rates of thoracentesis as compared to paracentesis, TIPS is preferred when possible over repeated thoracentesis for patients with refractory hepatic hydrothorax.

Spontaneous Bacterial Peritonitis

Spontaneous bacterial peritonitis (SBP) is an infection of the peritoneal fluid in the absence of a treatable surgical cause seen in patients with cirrhosis and ascites. It is thought to be caused by translocation of enteric bacteria.[22] The most common bacteria involved are gram-negative organisms (*Escherichia coli* and Klebsiella). The clinical picture is typically characterized by fever and/or hypothermia, abdominal pain and tenderness, and occasionally peripheral leukocytosis. Severe cases can lead to renal failure, hypotension, and shock. Up to 10% of the patients are asymptomatic, and therefore a high level of suspicion is necessary.

The diagnosis of SBP requires a diagnostic paracentesis with an elevated WBC count (>250 neutrophils per mL) and/or a positive ascites fluid culture. Culture-negative neutrocytic ascites (CNNA) is clinically indistinguishable from SBP except that no bacteria are grown on culture. CNNA should be treated the same as SBP.

The treatment of SBP includes antibiotic therapy and intravenous albumin. The antibiotic of choice is a third-generation cephalosporin and a 5-day course is usually sufficient. Oral fluoroquinolones can be considered for stable patients in hospitals or communities with low resistance to fluoroquinolones. A second diagnostic paracentesis 48 hours after initiation of therapy to document a decrease in PMNs and no growth is common practice although not currently part of the American Association for the Study of Liver Diseases

(AASLD) guidelines. If no response is seen, antibiotics should be changed and secondary bacterial peritonitis should be suspected.

Renal insufficiency develops in one-third of patients with SBP[23] and is associated with a high mortality. The incidence of renal dysfunction can be reduced by 30% and the 3-month mortality by 50% with the use of albumin 1.5 g/kg of body weight at diagnosis followed by 1 g/kg of body weight on day 3.[24] Seventy percent of patients with SBP will have a second episode of SBP within 1 year.[25] This can be reduced to 20% with secondary prophylaxis using norfloxacin 400 mg daily. Other fluoroquinolones or bactrim have also been used for secondary prophylaxis. Daily prophylaxis has been shown to be superior to weekly dosing and should be used in all cases.

Though more controversial, those patients who are at a high risk of developing SBP but have never experienced an episode are also likely to benefit from primary prophylaxis using the same regimen. This includes patients with low total protein in their ascites fluid (<1.5 g/dL) and signs of advanced liver disease (Child-Pugh score ≥9 with bilirubin >3 mg/dL), hyponatremia (serum sodium <130 mEq/L), or renal dysfunction.[26]

Hepatorenal Syndrome

Hepatorenal syndrome (HRS) is defined as renal insufficiency that occurs in the absence of intrinsic renal disease in patients with portal HTN. It is due to extreme renal artery vasoconstriction in setting of severe peripheral vasodilatation with extreme activation of RAAS. Figure 2-4 describes the evaluation and management in a patient with suspected HRS. It starts with a 25% albumin challenge, followed by ongoing albumin with therapy to lower portal pressures (octreotide or vasopressin/terlipressin) and increase systemic vascular resistance (midodrine or vasopressin/terlipressin). Terlipressin is a vasopressin analog currently approved in Europe for use in HRS. A large multicenter, randomized, double-blind, placebo-controlled study showed benefit with reversal of HRS in one-third of patients.[27] A second multicenter, randomized, placebo-controlled, phase III trial is currently underway[28] and could lead to the United States' approval of this agent. Since the outcomes are extremely poor, urgent transplant should be performed whenever possible for HRS in appropriate candidates and will result in reversal of renal failure when performed promptly.

Hepatic Encephalopathy

Definition, Pathogenesis, and Classification

Hepatic encephalopathy (HE) is a spectrum of neurocognitive and neuropsychiatric abnormalities seen in patients with portal HTN and/or

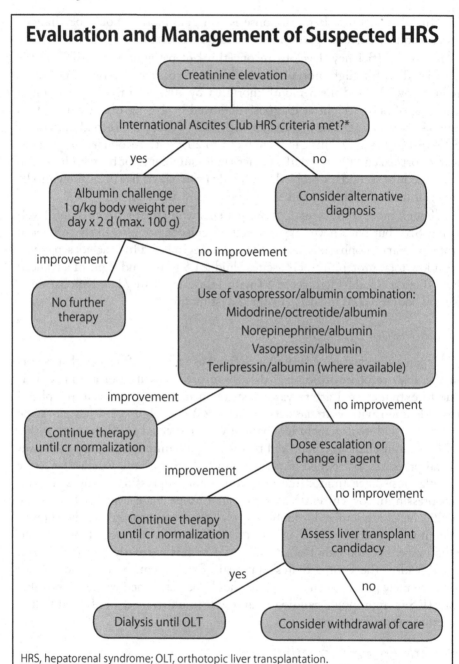

Figure 2-4. Evaluation and management of suspected HRS.

hepatic dysfunction. The pathophysiological basis of HE is still under debate, but low-grade cerebral edema, an effect of ammonia, and other toxin accumulation in the brain are leading theories.[30] Decreased hepatocyte mass and portosystemic shunting lead to higher levels of ammonia reaching the brain. Astrocytes, through glutamine synthetase, convert glutamine to glutamate, detoxifying ammonia in the process. The higher glutamine concentrations in the astrocytes raise the oncotic pressure causing water inflow and leading to "low-grade cerebral edema." Other known precipitants of hepatic encephalopathy have also been shown to cause astrocyte swelling such as hyponatremia, benzodiazepines, and inflammatory cytokines. Not visible in usual brain imaging, this low-grade edema can be detected with other techniques such as magnetic resonance spectroscopy (MRS) or magnetization transfer ratio (MTR).

HE can be classified as minimal (also termed *covert*) when the cognitive alterations are not clinically evident and need to be detected using neurophysiological or neuropsychological testing and overt HE, which can be diagnosed clinically.

Overt Hepatic Encephalopathy

The criteria used for diagnosis and the classification of HE has not changed in over 30 years. The West Haven criteria as modified by Conn are still used[31] (Table 2-3).[32]

HE is generally episodic following periods of increased ammonia levels (eg, gastrointestinal bleeding) or other known exacerbating factors of the low-grade cerebral edema (eg, infection, benzodiazepines, hyponatremia). Patients may or may not recover completely following episodes of HE.

The treatment of an acute episode of HE is aimed at treating the precipitating factor followed by therapies to lower ammonia levels. Since most of the ammonia in the circulation is produced by intestinal bacteria, most of the therapies for HE aim at reducing intestinal ammonia levels or absorption. The gold standard treatment is lactulose. Data on lactulose are scant and poor quality and a recent Cochrane database[33] questioned its value. A more recent randomized controlled trial showed a 50% efficacy in decreasing new episodes of HE in high-risk patients.[34]

For patients with recurrent episodes of HE, rifaximin should be considered to maintain remission. Rifaximin is a nonselective nonabsorbable antibiotic used as early as the 1980s in the treatment of HE. Approval by the FDA for secondary prevention of HE after large pivotal study including 300 patients with cirrhosis and a history of recurrent HE showed a 50% reduction in subsequent episodes of and hospitalizations for HE.[35] It is well tolerated with few side effects given its minimal absorption.

Other therapies that can be considered but are not approved by the FDA or considered standard of care include zinc, L-ornithine L-aspartate (LOLA), probiotics, or, in severe cases, albumin dialysis.

Table 2-3

West Haven Grading of Encephalopathy

NORMAL				
Minimal HE (Stage 0)	I	II	III	IV
West Haven Scale	Euphoria or anxiety Trivial lack of awareness Shortened attention span Impairment of ability to add or subtract	Lethargy or apathy Disorientation with respect to time Obvious personality change Inappropriate behavior	Somnolence or semi-stupor Confusion Responsiveness to stimuli Gross disorientation Bizarre behavior	Coma

Reproduced with permission from Ferenci P, Lockwood A, Mullen K, Tarter R, Weissenborn K, Blei AT. Hepatic encephalopathy--definition, nomenclature, diagnosis, and quantification: final report of the working party at the 11th World Congresses of Gastroenterology, Vienna, 1998. *Hepatology.* 2002;35(3):716-721.

Minimal Hepatic Encephalopathy

Minimal HE is defined as cognitive alterations seen on neuropsychological or neurophysiological testing in the absence of clinical signs or symptoms of HE. The prevalence is as high as 80% in some studies. Patients with minimal HE have a lower quality of life, lower work performance, driving impairments, and a higher risk of developing overt HE.[36] Screening patients with cirrhosis for minimal HE is not universally done mostly due to the absence of consensus on who should be screened, what battery of tests to use, and no clear guidelines on appropriate treatment. While many of the therapies used for overt HE such as lactulose, probiotics, LOLA, and poorly absorbable antibiotics have been shown to improve some measures of minimal HE, there is a lack of high-quality, randomized, placebo-controlled trials. The exception is the use of rifaximin, with a recent large randomized, placebo-controlled trial showing higher resolution rates and improved quality of life.[37] The significant cost of rifaximin is a concern for long-term use in this very prevalent complication of cirrhosis.

Pulmonary Complications

Two poorly understood pulmonary complications are seen in patients with cirrhosis, portal HTN, and hepatopulmonary and portopulmonary syndromes.

Hepatopulmonary Syndrome

Hepatopulmonary syndrome is a hypoxic condition caused by intrapulmonary shunting. Patients experience shortness of breath, decreased exercise capacity, and platypnea-orthodeoxia (desaturation and dyspnea in upright position that improve by supine positioning). Its diagnosis requires proof of alveolar-arterial O_2 gradient and the presence of intrapulmonary vascular dilatations as seen by bubble echocardiogram, technetium labeled macroaggregated albumin scanning, or pulmonary angiography. Estimated incidence is 4% to 29% in patients with cirrhosis.[38] The only treatment is oxygen supplementation to prevent pulmonary hypertension and liver transplantation, which reverses the condition.

Portopulmonary Syndrome

Portopulmonary syndrome is a pulmonary HTN seen in patients with portal HTN. Right heart catheterization is used for diagnosis. The estimated incidence is 2% to 10%.[38] The treatment is similar to primary pulmonary HTN with use of pulmonary vasodilators such as prostacyclin, oral endothelin receptor antagonists, or phosphodiesterase inhibitors. Patients should be referred to specialized liver transplant centers due to the high perioperative morbidity and mortality seen. This condition stabilizes but does not always reverse with transplantation.

SPECIAL ISSUES IN HEALTH CARE MAINTENANCE

Patients with cirrhosis have coagulation abnormalities with prolongation of their prothrombin time (PT) and partial thromboplastin time (PTT) as well as thrombocytopenia due to splachnic sequestration. These coagulation abnormalities are due to a decreased production of coagulation factors in the liver (all coagulation factors except factor VIII). Anticoagulants are also produced in the liver and reduced. The prolongation in PT is not an accurate predictor of bleeding risk. In general, low-risk procedures such as endoscopies and colonoscopies without intervention (no polypectomy, no biopsies) and paracentesis can be performed without replacement of factors or platelets. Those procedures that have a higher risk of bleeding such as thoracentesis, liver biopsy, or polypectomy should be performed with adequate replacement of factors and platelets. Eltrombopag, an oral thrombopoietin-receptor agonist that stimulates thrombopoiesis and elevates platelet count, was shown to be effective in raising platelet counts in patients with HCV-related cirrhosis, increasing the number of patients that were able to initiate therapy with pegylated interferon and ribavirin.[39] A multicenter, randomized, double-blind, placebo-controlled phase III trial looking at reduction in platelet transfusion needs in patients with cirrhosis undergoing elective procedures is currently underway.[28]

REFERENCES

1. Dufour MC. Chronic liver disease and cirrhosis. In: Everhart JE, ed. Digestive diseases in the United States: epidemiology and impact. US Department of Health and Human Services, Public Health Service, National Institutes of Health, National Institute of Diabetes and Digestive and Kidney Diseases. Washington, DC: US Government Printing Office. 1994;94-1447:613–646.

2. Heron M. Deaths: leading causes for 2007. *Natl Vital Stat Rep.* 2011;59(8):1-95.

3. Ghany MG, Strader DB, Thomas DL, Seeff LB. Diagnosis, management, and treatment of hepatitis C: an update. *Hepatology.* 2009;49(4):1335-1374.

4. Gines P, Quintero E, Arroyo V, et al. Compensated cirrhosis: natural history and prognostic factors. *Hepatology.* 1987;7(1):122-128.

5. Pugh RN, Murray-Lyon IM, Dawson JL, Pietroni MC, Williams R. Transection of the oesophagus for bleeding oesophageal varices. *Br J Surg.* 1973;60(8):646-649.

6. Malinchoc M, Kamath PS, Gordon FD, Peine CJ, Rank J, ter Borg PC. A model to predict poor survival in patients undergoing transjugular intrahepatic portosystemic shunts. *Hepatology.* 2000;31(4):864-871.

7. Organ Procurement and Transplantation Network (OPTN) and Scientific Registry of Transplant Recipients (SRTR). OPTN/SRTR 2010 Annual Data Report. Rockville, MD: Department of Health and Human Services, Health Resources and Services Administration, Healthcare Systems Bureau, Division of Transplantation; 2011:9-143.

8. Merion RM, Schaubel DE, Dykstra DM, Freeman RB, Port FK, Wolfe RA. The survival benefit of liver transplantation. *Am J Transplant.* 2005;5(2):307-313.

9. Schaubel DE, Sima CS, Goodrich NP, Feng S, Merion RM. The survival benefit of deceased donor liver transplantation as a function of candidate disease severity and donor quality. *Am J Transplant.* 2008;8(2):419-425.

10. Sanyal AJ, Bosch J, Blei A, Arroyo V. Portal hypertension and its complications. *Gastroenterology.* 2008;134(6):1715-1728.

11. Runyon BA. Management of adult patients with ascites due to cirrhosis: an update. *Hepatology.* 2009;49(6):2087-2107.

12. Garcia-Tsao G, Sanyal AJ, Grace ND, Carey W. Prevention and management of gastroesophageal varices and variceal hemorrhage in cirrhosis. *Hepatology.* 2007;46(3):922-938.

13. EASL clinical practice guidelines on the management of ascites, spontaneous bacterial peritonitis, and hepatorenal syndrome in cirrhosis. *J Hepatol.* 2010;53(3):397-417.

14. Tripathi D, Ferguson JW, Kochar N, et al. Randomized controlled trial of carvedilol versus variceal band ligation for the prevention of the first variceal bleed. *Hepatology.* 2009;50(3):825-833.

15. Lebrec D, Poynard T, Hillon P, Benhamou JP. Propranolol for prevention of recurrent gastrointestinal bleeding in patients with cirrhosis: a controlled study. *N Engl J Med.* 1981;305(23):1371-1374.

16. Graham DY, Smith JL. The course of patients after variceal hemorrhage. *Gastroenterology.* 1981;80(4):800-809.

17. Garcia-Pagan JC, Caca K, Bureau C, et al. Early use of TIPS in patients with cirrhosis and variceal bleeding. *N Engl J Med.* 2010;362(25):2370-2379.

18. Ripoll C, Groszmann R, Garcia-Tsao G, et al. Hepatic venous pressure gradient predicts clinical decompensation in patients with compensated cirrhosis. *Gastroenterology.* 2007;133(2):481-488.

19. Gines P, Guevara M. Hyponatremia in cirrhosis: pathogenesis, clinical significance, and management. *Hepatology.* 2008;48(3):1002-1010.

20. Angeli P, Wong F, Watson H, Gines P. Hyponatremia in cirrhosis: results of a patient population survey. *Hepatology.* 2006;44(6):1535-1542.

21. O'Leary JG, Davis GL. Conivaptan increases serum sodium in hyponatremic patients with end-stage liver disease. *Liver Transpl.* 2009;15(10):1325-1329.

22. Cirera I, Bauer TM, Navasa M, et al. Bacterial translocation of enteric organisms in patients with cirrhosis. *J Hepatol.* 2001;34(1):32-37.

23. Follo A, Llovet JM, Navasa M, et al. Renal impairment after spontaneous bacterial peritonitis in cirrhosis: incidence, clinical course, predictive factors and prognosis. *Hepatology.* 1994;20(6):1495-1501.

24. Sort P, Navasa M, Arroyo V, et al. Effect of intravenous albumin on renal impairment and mortality in patients with cirrhosis and spontaneous bacterial peritonitis. *N Engl J Med.* 1999;341(6):403-409.

25. Tító L, Rimola A, Ginès P, Llach J, Arroyo V, Rodés J. Recurrence of spontaneous bacterial peritonitis in cirrhosis: frequency and predictive factors. *Hepatology.* 1988;8(1):27-31.

26. Fernandez J, Navasa M, Planas R, et al. Primary prophylaxis of spontaneous bacterial peritonitis delays hepatorenal syndrome and improves survival in cirrhosis. *Gastroenterology.* 2007;133(3):818-824.

27. Sanyal AJ, Boyer T, Garcia-Tsao G, et al. A randomized, prospective, double-blind, placebo-controlled trial of terlipressin for type 1 hepatorenal syndrome. *Gastroenterology.* 2008;134(5):1360-1368.

28. US National Institutes of Health. URL: http://www.clinicaltrials.gov/ct2/search. Search criteria: terlipressin, hepatorenal syndrome. Accessed December 2011.

29. International Club of Ascites. Criteria for the diagnosis of hepatorenal syndrome. URL: www. icascites.org/about/guidelines/. Accessed December 2011.

30. Haussinger D, Schliess F. Pathogenetic mechanisms of hepatic encephalopathy. *Gut.* 2008;57(8):1156-1165.

31. Atterbury CE, Maddrey WC, Conn HO. Neomycin-sorbitol and lactulose in the treatment of acute portal-systemic encephalopathy. A controlled, double-blind clinical trial. *Am J Dig Dis.* 1978;23(5):398-406.

32. Ferenci P, Lockwood A, Mullen K, Tarter R, Weissenborn K, Blei AT. Hepatic encephalopathy--definition, nomenclature, diagnosis, and quantification: final report of the working party at the 11th World Congresses of Gastroenterology, Vienna, 1998. *Hepatology.* 2002;35(3):716-721.

33. Als-Nielsen B, Gluud LL, Gluud C. Nonabsorbable disaccharides for hepatic encephalopathy. *Cochrane Database Syst Rev.* 2004(2):CD003044.

34. Sharma BC, Sharma P, Agrawal A, Sarin SK. Secondary prophylaxis of hepatic encephalopathy: an open-label randomized controlled trial of lactulose versus placebo. *Gastroenterology.* 2009;137(3):885-891, 891 e881.

35. Bass NM, Mullen KD, Sanyal A, et al. Rifaximin treatment in hepatic encephalopathy. *N Engl J Med.* 2010;362(12):1071-1081.

36. Montgomery JY, Bajaj JS. Advances in the evaluation and management of minimal hepatic encephalopathy. *Curr Gastroenterol Rep.* 2011;13(1):26-33.

37. Sidhu SS, Goyal O, Mishra BP, Sood A, Chhina RS, Soni RK. Rifaximin improves psychometric performance and health-related quality of life in patients with minimal hepatic encephalopathy (the RIME Trial). *Am J Gastroenterol.* 2011;106(2):307-316.

38. Hoeper MM, Krowka MJ, Strassburg CP. Portopulmonary hypertension and hepatopulmonary syndrome. *Lancet.* 2004;363(9419):1461-1468.

39. McHutchison JG, Dusheiko G, Shiffman ML, et al. Eltrombopag for thrombocytopenia in patients with cirrhosis associated with hepatitis C. *N Engl J Med.* 2007;357(22):2227-2236.

3

Hepatocellular Carcinoma and Cholangiocarcinoma

Mark W. Russo, MD, MPH, FACG, AGAF

HEPATOCELLULAR CARCINOMA

Epidemiology

Regardless of etiology, all patients with cirrhosis are at risk for hepatocellular carcinoma (HCC). For patients with chronic hepatitis B, screening should be performed even if the patient does not have cirrhosis. HCC is the fifth leading cause of death from cancer in men worldwide and seventh in women with more than 700,000 cases worldwide in 2008.[1] In the United States it is estimated that HCC will occur in 28,000 individuals and account for more than 20,000 deaths.[2] In 2007, there were approximately 27,753 individuals who had cancer of the liver or intrahepatic bile ducts.[2] Twice as many men were affected as women. Cirrhosis from viral hepatitis is one of the major risk factors for HCC. The risk of HCC in hepatitis C cirrhosis is estimated to be 4.8% over a mean of 4.6 years, but even patients with cirrhosis from nonalcoholic fatty liver disease (NAFLD) are at increased risk for HCC.[3,4] Because of the obesity epidemic and the increasing number of patients with cirrhosis from NAFLD, the rate of HCC is likely to increase over the next decade.

Patients with cirrhosis, especially those awaiting liver transplantation, should undergo screening and surveillance for HCC. Screening is a one-time

Brown RS Jr. *Common Liver Diseases and Transplantation:
An Algorithmic Approach to Work-Up and Management (pp 35-45).*
© 2013 Taylor & Francis Group.

Table 3-1

Proposed Surveillance for Hepatocellular Carcinoma

- Ultrasound every 6 months with or without AFP.
- Some centers may alternate ultrasound with CT abdomen triple phase or MRI abdomen with IV contrast every 6 months, such as patients listed for liver transplant.

*Patients who have chronic hepatitis B without cirrhosis should also undergo screening for HCC.

AFP, alpha-fetoprotein; CT, computed tomography; MRI, magnetic resonance imaging; HCC, hepatocellular carcinoma.

evaluation for cancer while surveillance indicates ongoing evaluation for cancer. Here, the term *screening* will be used to indicate both terms. Patients with cirrhosis from alcohol, viral hepatitis, NAFLD, and hemochromatosis are at the greatest risk for HCC when compared to patients with cirrhosis from alpha-1-antitrypsin deficiency, autoimmune liver disease, primary biliary cirrhosis, or primary sclerosing cholangitis. According to the recent American Association for the Study of Liver Diseases (AASLD) guidelines, all patients with a diagnosis of cirrhosis should undergo a transabdominal ultrasound of the liver every 6 months.[5] Alpha-fetoprotein (AFP) is no longer recommended by the AASLD for screening unless imaging is unavailable, but it is still used by many experts. Though high levels of AFP are quite specific for HCC, AFP is not a sensitive test so normal levels should not replace imaging. Our screening schedule for HCC is shown in Table 3-1.[6]

Diagnosis and Work-Up of Hepatocellular Carcinoma

HCC may be detected incidentally or during screening. If a suspicious lesion is seen on ultrasound, a cross-sectional imaging study, such as a computed tomography (CT) scan or magnetic resonance imaging (MRI) of the abdomen, should be obtained with intravenous contrast. Patients with lesions that have classic findings for HCC on imaging may not require a biopsy of the lesion (Figure 3-1). The appropriate liver imaging is a 4-phase CT of the abdomen or MRI of the abdomen with IV contrast that includes an arterial phase, portal phase, and delayed (including equilibrium and venous) phase (Table 3-2). Classic findings for HCC on imaging with CT or MRI include late arterial enhancement, rapid washout during the portal venous phases, and peripheral rim enhancement on the delayed phase.[7] New criteria for listing patients with Model End-Stage Liver Disease (MELD) exception

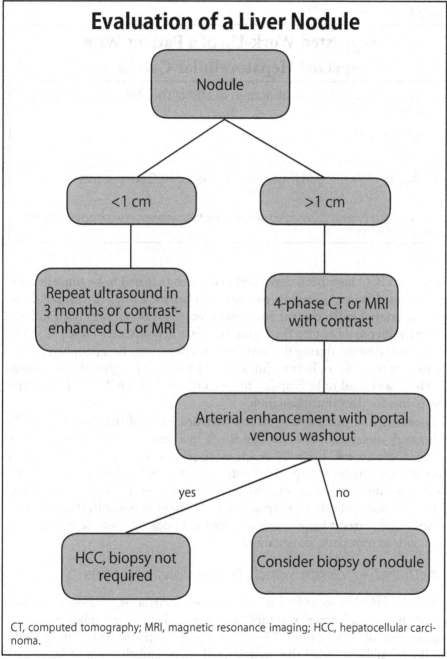

Figure 3-1. Evaluation of a liver nodule discovered on ultrasound in a cirrhotic patient. (Adapted from Bruix J, Sherman M. Management of hepatocellular carcinoma. *Hepatology.* 2010;53:1-35.)

Table 3-2

Suggested Work-Up of a Patient With
Suspected Hepatocellular Carcinoma

- Triple-phase CT of the abdomen or MRI of the abdomen with IV contrast
- CT of the chest
- AFP
- Biopsy of liver lesion if imaging criteria for HCC are not met

AFP, alpha-fetoprotein; CT, computed tomography; MRI, magnetic resonance imaging; HCC, hepatocellular carcinoma.

points for HCC have been developed and are anticipated to be implemented in the United States.[7] Cirrhotic patients with hepatic lesions that do not demonstrate arterial enhancement with portal venous washout may need to have the lesion biopsied because the lesion may be a hypovascular HCC. A lesion that retains contrast during the portal venous phase may be a peripheral cholangiocarcinoma. Thus, liver nodules that do not meet imaging characteristics for HCC will need to be biopsied to be considered for HCC MELD exception points for liver transplantation.

Assessment of extrahepatic disease includes a CT of the chest to exclude pulmonary metastases. A bone scan is not routinely ordered unless a patient has focal symptoms. Enlarged reactive lymph nodes are commonly seen in patients with cirrhosis, especially patients with viral hepatitis and autoimmune liver disease, but an enlarging lymph node or a lymph node greater than 3 cm may indicate metastatic disease. Lymph nodes with these characteristics may warrant biopsy (percutaneous or endoscopic ultrasound guided) to exclude extrahepatic malignant disease.

Treatment Algorithms and Special Considerations

Once a HCC is identified in a patient with cirrhosis, treatment options include resection, locoregional therapy, systemic therapy, transplantation, or a combination of these options. There is no standard approach to treating HCC but it can safely be stated that transarterial chemoembolization (TACE) and percutaneous ablation (using radiofrequency or microwave probes) are among the more common modalities used to treat patients with HCC. TACE has been shown in a randomized trial to improve survival.[8] Because fewer than

Table 3-3

Common Treatment Options for
Hepatocellular Carcinoma

- Transarterial chemoembolization
- Percutaneous or laparoscopic ablation radiofrequency, microwave, or cryotherapy
- Yttrium-90 radioembolization
- Systemic therapy (eg, sorafenib)
- Resection
- Transplantation

20% of cirrhotic patients are resection candidates, most patients undergo multimodality therapy that includes locoregional therapy with or without systemic therapy (Table 3-3).[6] Patients with single tumors up to 5 cm can undergo ablation therapy with radiofrequency or microwave ablation. Patients with multiple tumors may be candidates for TACE. TACE has the benefit of treating a region of liver supplied by the artery that is embolized, which is termed a *field effect*. Patients may undergo TACE followed by ablation. If patients are transplant candidates and their tumor falls within transplant criteria, they may undergo ablation or chemoembolization while they are undergoing evaluation or waiting ("bridged") to liver transplant. Tumors larger than 5 cm may be considered for yttrium-90 (radioembolization). A proposed treatment algorithm is shown in Figure 3-2.

Important factors to consider when determining if a patient is a candidate for locoregional therapy are the stage of cirrhosis and tumor burden. Patients with ascites, impaired renal function, and tumors greater than 5 to 10 cm may either be at risk for decompensating after ablation or TACE or may not derive a clinical benefit. Patients with a total serum bilirubin greater than 3 mg/dL may be at an increased risk for decompensation after TACE, but subselective embolization or ablation may be performed in select patients with elevated total bilirubin.

Sorafenib is the first systemic therapy to demonstrate a survival benefit in patients with unresectable HCC, although the benefit is modest with a 2.8-month survival advantage.[9] The advent of molecular markers and a better understanding of the pathogenesis of HCC have resulted in the developing targeted therapies against an otherwise resistant tumor.[10] Referring clinicians should contact nearby tertiary centers because there may be ongoing clinical trials for HCC.

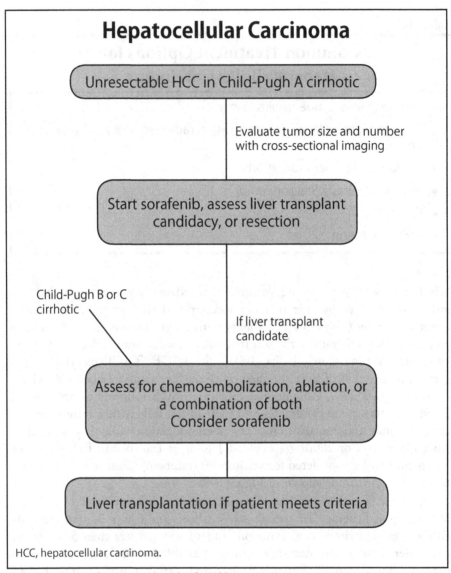

Figure 3-2. Proposed treatment algorithm for HCC.

Table 3-4

Hepatocellular Carcinoma That May Qualify for MELD Exception Points for Liver Transplantation

- Milan Criteria (national policy)
  - One nodule 2.0 to 5.0 cm
  - Two or 3 nodules all <3.0 cm
- UCSF Criteria (depends on regional policy)
  - One lesion >5 cm and up to 8 cm
  - Two to 3 lesions with at least one lesion >3 cm and not exceeding 5 cm, with total tumor diameter up to 8 cm
  - Four to 5 lesions with none >3 cm, with total tumor diameter up to 8 cm
  - Minimum waiting time of 3 months after downstaging
  - No vascular invasion on imaging studies

MELD, Model for End-Stage Liver Disease; UCSF, University of California San Francisco.

Patients with cirrhosis who develop HCC and who are not candidates for resection may receive additional priority for liver transplantation and transplant may be curative. In the United States, patients who meet the Milan (or Mazzaferro) criteria for HCC (one lesion ≤5 cm or ≤3 lesions ≤3 cm each) can receive a MELD score of 22, which is associated with a 3-month mortality of 15% and is increased every 3 months on the waiting list (Table 3-4). The 5-year survival after liver transplantation for HCC is approximately 75%. Tumors beyond these criteria can also receive transplant particularly if they are downstaged with locoregional therapy, but local practices vary and they may not receive additional priority for transplantation.

When to Refer Difficult Cases

Difficult cases usually include patients with advanced HCC, either large tumors or tumors invading the portal or hepatic veins, or patients with advanced cirrhosis. Suggested indications for referral are shown in Table 3-5.

Downstaging

Patients with HCC beyond the Milan criteria can be transplanted with acceptable outcomes. Patients who have tumors within the University of

Table 3-5

When to Refer a Patient With Hepatocellular Carcinoma

- Transplant evaluation
- TACE, ablation if not available locally
- Portal or hepatic vein invasion
- Child-Pugh class B or C cirrhosis, MELD score >20
- Patients outside Milan criteria but within UCSF criteria to determine if candidates for downstaging

TACE, transarterial chemoembolization; MELD, Model for End-Stage Liver Disease; UCSF, University of California San Francisco.

California San Francisco (UCSF) criteria (see Table 3-4) have post-transplant patient survival similar to patients transplanted under the Milan criteria.[11] Patients with HCC that meet UCSF criteria may be treated with locoregional or multimodality therapy. If the patient's tumor burden falls within Milan criteria on subsequent cross-sectional imaging, the tumor may be considered "downstaged." Some centers may offer patients liver transplant after the patient is considered downstaged for a defined period of time, typically 3 to 6 months. Patients who develop tumors that grow beyond Milan criteria after successful downstaging may have aggressive tumors. These patients are at high risk for recurrence of HCC after transplant and may not be suitable liver transplant candidates.

CHOLANGIOCARCINOMA

In contrast to the more common liver diseases such as viral hepatitis and alcoholic liver disease, which are associated with an increased risk of HCC, patients with primary sclerosing cholangitis (PSC) are predisposed to developing cholangiocarcinoma. However, only 20% of cholangiocarcinomas occur in patients with PSC. Unfortunately, screening methods for cholangiocarcinoma are of unproven benefit, including CA 19-9, endoscopic biopsies, and brushing of the biliary tree.[12,13] A CA 19-9 value of more than 100 U/mL has a sensitivity of only 75% and values over 100 U/mL are not specific for cholangiocarcinoma.[12] The positive predictive value of cytology from bile duct brushings is 68% for cholangiocarcinoma.[13] One unproven approach is to image patients with PSC with abdominal MRI

Table 3-6

Treatment Options for Cholangiocarcinoma

- Resection
- Chemotherapy-gemcitabine ± radiation therapy
- Liver transplantation

so magnetic resonance cholangiopancreatography (MRCP) images could be obtained during the evaluation to look for cholangiocarcinoma. Although MRCP is excellent in delineating the extrahepatic biliary system, its role in screening for cholangiocarcinoma has not been proven to be beneficial.[14]

Treatment of cholangiocarcinoma is challenging because it is resistant to chemotherapy and radiation and few patients benefit from resection (Table 3-6). In carefully selected patients with cholangiocarcinoma, acceptable long-term outcomes have been reported from a single center series of patients who were treated with neoadjuvant chemoradiation and pretransplant staging exploratory laparotomy[15] (Table 3-7). The Mayo Clinic protocol for liver transplant candidates with cholangiocarcinoma includes external beam radiation and 5-fluorouracil for 3 weeks followed by brachytherapy for 2 weeks. Capecitabine is administered until the time of transplantation. Abdominal exploration for staging is performed near time of anticipated deceased donor transplantation or the day prior to living donor transplantation. The Mayo Clinic has reported results in 120 patients who underwent liver transplantation for cholangiocarcinoma. Five-year survival after liver transplantation is 73%.[15] Before EUS was used for staging, 40% to 50% of patients did not proceed with liver transplant due to findings at staging operation. After EUS with aspiration of regional lymph nodes was implemented, less than 15% of patients are excluded due to findings during the staging operation. Thus, carefully selected patients with cholangiocarcinoma who undergo neoadjuvant chemoradiation with staging exploratory laparotomy have good long-term post-transplant survival rates, but these patients should be managed at centers experienced with protocols for cholangiocarcinoma.

SUMMARY

Effective treatment for HCC in cirrhotic patients includes a multimodality approach with locoregional therapy, systemic therapy, and in select cases

Table 3-7

Potential Liver Transplant Candidates With Cholangiocarcinoma

- Unresectable tumor above cystic duct or resectable in setting of PSC
- Transcatheter biopsy or brush cytology
- CA 19-9 >100 U/mL and/or a mass on cross-sectional imaging and malignant stricture on cholangiogram
- Biliary aneuploidy on FISH with malignant appearing stricture on cholangiogram
- Radial tumor diameter <3 cm
- Absence of intra- and extrahepatic disease
- No history of prior radiation or chemotherapy
- No history of prior biliary resection or attempt at resection
- No history of transperitoneal biopsy either percutaneous or EUS FNA

FISH, fluorescent in situ hybridization; PSC, primary sclerosing cholangitis; CA, carbohydrate antigen; EUS, endoscopic ultrasound; FNA, fine needle aspirate. (Adapted from Rosen CB, Heimbach JK, Gores GJ. Liver transplantation for cholangiocarcinoma. *Transpl Int.* 2010;23(7):692-697.)

liver transplantation. Resection can be considered in select patients with early cirrhosis who have small left-sided lesions or lesions near the capsule. Cholangiocarcinoma is more difficult to treat, and patients should be considered for resection. A small group of patients may be eligible for liver transplantation and post-transplant survival is excellent in this select group. Future therapy is likely to be guided by molecular markers targeting tumor pathways.

REFERENCES

1. Global Cancer: Facts and Figures. 2nd ed. American Cancer Society. Atlanta, GA. URL: http://www.cancer.org/acs/groups/content/@epidemiologysurveilance/documents/document/acspc-027766.pdf. Accessed July 5, 2012.

2. National Cancer Institute. SEER Stat Fact Sheets: Liver and Intrahepatic Bile Duct. URL: http://seer.cancer.gov/statfacts/html/livibd.html. Accessed July 5 2012.

3. Lok AS, Seeff LB, Morgan TR, et al. Incidence of hepatocellular carcinoma and associated risk factors in hepatitis C-related advanced liver disease. *Gastroenterology.* 2009;136(1):138-148.

4. Starley BQ, Calcagno CJ, Harrison SA. Nonalcoholic fatty liver disease and hepatocellular carcinoma: a weighty connection. *Hepatology.* 2010;51(5):1820-1832.

5. American Association for the Study of Liver Diseases. Alexandria, VA. URL: http://www. AASLD.org. Accessed July 10, 2012.

6. Bruix J, Sherman M. Management of hepatocellular carcinoma. *Hepatology.* 2010;53:1-35.

7. Pomfret EA, Washburn K, Wald C, et al. Report of a national conference on liver allocation in patients with hepatocellular carcinoma. *Liver Transpl.* 2010;16(3):262-278.

8. Llovet JM, Bruix J. Systematic review of randomized trials for unresectable hepatocellular carcinoma: chemoembolization improves survival. *Hepatology.* 2003;37(2):429-442.

9. Llovet JM, Ricci S, Mazzaferro V, et al. Sorafenib in advanced hepatocellular carcinoma. *New Engl J Med.* 2008;359(4):378-390.

10. Siegel AB, Olsen SK, Magun A, Brown RS Jr. Sorafenib: where do we go from here? *Hepatology.* 2010;52(1):360-369.

11. Yao FY, Hirose R, LaBerge JM, et al. A prospective study on downstaging of hepatocellular carcinoma prior to liver transplantation. *Liver Transpl.* 2005;11(12):1505-1514.

12. Singh P, Patel T. Advances in the diagnosis, evaluation and management of cholangiocarcinoma. *Curr Opin Gastroenterol.* 2006;22(3):294-299.

13. Boberg KM, Jebsen P, Clausen OP, Foss A, Aabakken L, Schrumpf E. Diagnostic benefit of biliary brush cytology in cholangiocarcinoma in primary sclerosing cholangitis. *J Hepatol.* 2006;45(4):568-574.

14. Manfredi R, Barbaro B, Masselli G, Vecchioli A, Marano P. Magnetic resonance imaging of cholangiocarcinoma. *Semin Liver Dis.* 2004;24(2):155-164.

15. Rosen CB, Heimbach JK, Gores GJ. Liver transplantation for cholangiocarcinoma. *Transpl Int.* 2010;23(7):692-697.

4

Evaluation of the Transplant Candidate

Mark W. Russo, MD, MPH, FACG, AGAF

Candidates for liver transplantation undergo a thorough medical, surgical, psychosocial, and financial evaluation prior to listing for transplantation. The Model for End-Stage Liver Disease (MELD) is used to prioritize patients for liver transplantation with the fundamental concept of giving organs to the sickest first. The MELD score is calculated based on serum total bilirubin, creatinine, and international normalized ratio. However, exceptions exist, such as patients with hepatocellular carcinoma who are within Milan criteria. Because of the organ shortage and wait list mortality in many areas of the country, strategies have been developed to expand the donor pool, including donation after cardiac death, extended criteria donors, and living donor donation. Effective management of potential complications that may develop including spontaneous bacterial peritonitis, variceal bleeding, encephalopathy, and hepatocellular carcinoma is crucial so patients can survive until they are transplanted. Effective communication and coordination of care between the transplant center and referring physician can help reduce the burden placed upon the patient and more efficiently deliver care.

Brown RS Jr. *Common Liver Diseases and Transplantation:*
An Algorithmic Approach to Work-Up and Management (pp 47-63).
© 2013 Taylor & Francis Group.

INTRODUCTION

There are 16,795 individuals waiting for a liver transplant and 1592 patients died waiting in 2011.[1] Most patients awaiting liver transplant are co-managed between their referring gastroenterologist or clinician and the transplant center. Effective communication and an understanding of when and where testing and follow-up is provided are fundamental to providing good care to the patient. The focus of this chapter is to discuss how patients awaiting liver transplantation can be successfully managed between their referring clinician and the transplant center.

Since February 2002, the MELD score has been used to allocate organs. MELD is more objective and at least equally effective in identifying patients at highest risk for mortality compared to the Child-Turcotte-Pugh (CTP) score.[2] Prior to 2002 livers were allocated by the United Network for Organ Sharing (UNOS) using a status code (2-3), which incorporated the CTP score. The CTP score contains factors that may have a subjective interpretation, such as the amount of ascites or degree of encephalopathy. In addition, the CTP score may have a ceiling effect because the highest score a patient can receive is 15. Thus, a patient with a serum total bilirubin of 14 mg/dL with elevated international normalized ratio (INR) and moderate ascites may receive a CTP of 15 as would a patient with a bilirubin of 4 mg/dL with the same INR and amount of ascites.

TRANSPLANT EVALUATION

Guidelines are published that suggest when a patient with cirrhosis should be evaluated for liver transplant (Table 4-1).[3] In general, once the MELD score is 10 or higher or significant signs of hepatic decompensation occur, patients should be referred for liver transplant. There are less common indications for referral including hepatopulmonary syndrome, portopulmonary hypertension, primary amyloidosis, primary oxalosis, or early stage cholangiocarcinoma, but these patients should be discussed between the referring clinician and transplant hepatologist (Table 4-2).[4]

The timing of when a patient should be referred for transplant may vary by region of the country because of differences in waiting time and MELD score at the time of liver transplant. For example, in the Northeast the mean MELD score at time of transplant is higher compared to the Southeast. Thus, the MELD score at the time a liver transplant evaluation is initiated may be higher at some programs in New York compared to Charlotte. A reasonable approach is to refer or call the transplant center once a patient develops decompensated liver disease and a MELD score higher than 10.

Table 4-1

Proposed Common Indications for Referring a Cirrhotic Patient for Liver Transplant Evaluation

- MELD >12
- Ascites requiring diuretics
- Recurrent variceal hemorrhage
- Encephalopathy requiring lactulose
- Hepatocellular carcinoma within transplant criteria

Table 4-2

Examples of Conditions That May Be Granted MELD Exception Points

- Hepatocellular carcinoma within transplant criteria
- Cholangiocarcinoma within transplant criteria
- Hyponatremia
- Hepatopulmonary syndrome (room air PO_2 <60 mm Hg, but usually >50 mm Hg)
- Portopulmonary syndrome

Steps in Liver Transplant Evaluation

The liver transplant evaluation consists of the following components: medical evaluation, surgical evaluation, psychosocial evaluation, and financial evaluation. The order in which appointments and testing are scheduled varies across transplant centers. One approach is to initiate a transplant evaluation by referral to a transplant hepatologist who serves as the gatekeeper and triages new patients for the transplant center. A patient whose liver disease is partly or fully due to alcohol may require substance abuse counseling and may not be eligible to begin liver transplant evaluation until counseling is complete, or at least until some assurance that abstinence can be achieved. Once the hepatologist determines that a patient should proceed with liver transplant evaluation, then a financial counselor at the transplant center determines if and where the patient has transplant benefits. Some insurance carriers require that a patient be referred to a specific in-network center. Health plans may have a cap on transplant coverage or coverage for medication. After financial clearance, patients meet a liver transplant coordinator who may be a nurse with specialized training in transplantation and a transplant social worker. Next they are scheduled for medical testing (Table 4-3). After medical testing, patients are seen by a transplant surgeon. The patient is then presented to the liver selection committee, which may include all or some of the following professionals: hepatologists, transplant surgeons, social workers, psychologists or psychiatrists, nutritionists, pharmacists, financial counselors, and ethicists. If the committee believes the patient is a transplant candidate, then his or her "transplant packet" is submitted to his or her insurance company for approval to list and cover the transplant. Once the transplant center receives approval from the patient's insurance company, the patient is listed for liver transplant. Blood work for MELD score is obtained on the day of listing. Evaluation practices differ between transplant centers, and having a working relationship with a transplant center can expedite evaluation for your patients.

Much of the diagnostic testing ordered for liver transplant evaluation is performed to exclude cardiovascular or pulmonary disease or malignancy. Most, but not all, of the testing is typically done at the transplant center, but some of the tests may be obtained near the patient's home (see Table 4-3).

One approach to coordinate testing is to provide the patient with a list of tests he or she will have performed at the transplant center and tests he or she need to arrange through his or her provider at home. For example, cardiac testing, consultation with a cardiologist, and abdominal imaging occur at the transplant center, and upper endoscopy, colonoscopy, and immunizations can be arranged near the patient's home.

The process to evaluate and then list a patient for liver transplant may take several days to several months depending on the clinical circumstances. Liver transplant programs may have accelerated liver transplant evaluation pathways so that patients with high MELD scores, greater than 20 or 25 for example, can be evaluated within 2 to 3 weeks of presentation. Patients who present with acute liver failure are an exception because their mortality is very high and they are inpatients. These patients can be evaluated and listed within 24 hours in most cases. The transplant evaluation is geared toward identifying appropriate candidates for transplant who will benefit from the procedure. Given the shortage of organs, it also attempts to identify barriers to successful long-term outcome. Contraindications to transplant are included in Table 4-4 and Table 4-5. Because each transplant takes a limited resource from a too-large pool of patients at risk, societal benefit is maximized only if expected results are reasonable, usually defined as 1-year survival >70% and 5-year survival >50%.

Table 4-3

Typical Transplant Evaluation

TEST	REASON AND PLACE WHERE IT IS USUALLY PERFORMED
Abdominal CT (triple phase with and without contrast) or MRI (with and without gadolinium)	Exclude hepatocellular carcinoma, portal vein thrombosis, and obtain hepatic arterial anatomy; at least one scan usually obtained at transplant center Follow-up for HCC surveillance can be performed near patient's home
Pulmonary function tests, arterial blood gas	Exclude unrecognized obstructive or restrictive lung disease Transplant center or near patient's home
Echocardiogram with bubble study	Exclude valvular heart disease and left ventricular dysfunction, screen for pulmonary hypertension and hepatopulmonary syndrome Transplant center
EKG	Screen for cardiac arrhythmias Transplant center or near patient's home
Dobutamine echocardiogram or nuclear cardiac stress test or left heart catheterization	Screen for coronary artery disease Transplant center
Right heart catheterization	Confirmatory test in patients with echocardiograms suggestive of pulmonary hypertension Transplant center
Upper endoscopy	Screen for varices Patient's local gastroenterologist
Colonoscopy (patients >50 years old) or patients with PSC and ulcerative colitis	Screen for colorectal cancer Patient's local gastroenterologist

(continued)

Table 4-3 *(continued)*

Typical Transplant Evaluation

TEST	REASON AND PLACE WHERE IT IS USUALLY PERFORMED
Mammography (women >40 years old)	Screen for breast cancer Near patient's home
PPD	Screen for tuberculosis Near patient's home
Chest x-ray	Baseline exam for comparison Transplant center
Dental exam	Evaluate for active dental infection Transplant center or near patient's home
Bone densitometry	Screen for osteopenia/osteoporosis Transplant center or near patient's home

CT, computed tomography; HCC, hepatocellular carcinoma; EKG, electrocardiogram; PSC, primary sclerosing cholangitis; PPD, purified protein derivative.

Table 4-4

Contraindications to Liver Transplantation

MEDICAL
• Sepsis or uncontrolled infection
• Severe pulmonary hypertension (mean pulmonary pressure >35 mm Hg, systolic >60 mm Hg)
• Severe pulmonary fibrosis or COPD
• Symptomatic coronary artery disease
• Severe congestive heart failure
• Extrahepatic malignancy (except for nonmelanoma skin cancer)
• Peripheral cholangiocarcinoma (select hilar cholangiocarcinomas may be transplant eligible)

(continued)

Table 4-4 *(continued)*

Contraindications to Liver Transplantation

MEDICAL
• Irreversible neurological disease
• Malignancy (excluding nonmelanoma skin cancers, HCC, and cholangiocarcinoma that meet transplant criteria)
• AIDS
• Diseases that cannot be fixed by a transplant or that will make the surgery too high-risk
PSYCHOSOCIAL
• Inadequate financial coverage
• Uncontrolled psychiatric disease
• Inadequate social support
• Ongoing substance abuse or failure to complete an intensive outpatient program
SURGICAL
• Complete thrombosis of portal vein and superior mesenteric vein (few centers may offer transplant to these patients)

Table 4-5

Relative Contraindications to Liver Transplantation

• Cholangiocarcinoma
• Age > 25
• HIV seropositivity

PSYCHOSOCIAL EVALUATION

Psychosocial contraindications are a major reason for denying a patient liver transplantation. Ongoing substance abuse, including alcohol, marijuana, or cocaine, are some of the more common contraindications for liver transplantation. Many liver transplant centers in the United States require a defined period of abstinence, 6 months being the most common, and participation in a substance abuse counseling program.[5] A common frustration of referring clinicians and patients is that the transplant center does not clearly provide the criteria for substance abuse counseling. A general rule is that patients whose liver disease is all or partly due to alcohol and the last use was within 5 years of presentation should undergo an intensive outpatient program that is typically 90 hours and may take 3 to 6 months to complete. Acceptable programs can be found at http://findtreatment.samhsa.gov/. Alcoholics Anonymous (particularly with an identified sponsor) and church/religious support groups may meet the transplant center's requirements for substance abuse counseling if counseling and insight can be verified. Patients should undergo random monthly drug, alcohol, and nicotine screens. Centers may require patients abstain from nicotine products.

Despite the requirements for substance abuse counseling, 25% of patients who abused alcohol prior to liver transplantation will relapse after liver transplantation.[5] The precise duration of sobriety that is needed prior to transplant and the impact of relapse on graft survival is not well defined. A common approach is to require at least 6 months of abstinence and completion of a substance abuse counseling program with negative alcohol or urine toxicology screens. Patients with ongoing substance abuse as documented on positive serum alcohol or urine toxicology screens should not be considered for liver transplantation and listed patients may need to be removed from the liver transplant list. Patients should document an adequate social network capable of providing a combination of basic cares, including transportation, medication verification, and emotional support. Poor social support may be associated with noncompliance and poor outcomes after liver transplant. Patients with psychiatric disorders, such as depression or schizophrenia, should be treated and under the care of a mental health professional.

PRIORITY FOR LISTING

Livers are allocated to patients awaiting liver transplant by highest MELD score within each blood type. For example, a patient with blood type O and a MELD score of 24 is offered a blood type O liver before a patient with the same blood type and MELD score of 23. Waiting time is not accounted for in organ allocation unless patients have the same MELD score and blood type. Then the patient waiting *longer* at that MELD score is offered the organ first.

Patients with MELD scores of 17 or higher may derive a survival benefit with liver transplantation based upon an analysis of the Scientific Registry of Transplant Recipients (SRTR),[6] which collects data on all patients in the United States undergoing liver transplantation. The analysis demonstrates that the risk of mortality after liver transplantation is greater in patients with

MELD scores less than 15 compared to the risk of death without a liver transplant. The risk of death at 1 year with transplant is equal to the risk of death without transplant in cirrhotic patients with MELD scores from 15 to 17 and a clear survival benefit with transplant is seen in cirrhotic patients with MELD scores 18 and higher. Though there is no short-term benefit to patients with lower MELD scores due to the risk of the transplant operation, they may achieve long-term survival benefit and this should be determined on a case-by-case basis.

MELD score is determined by blood work but there are some notable exceptions where patients may receive a higher MELD score than what their blood work indicates. A patient with cirrhosis and unresectable hepatocellular carcinoma within certain (Milan) criteria may receive a MELD score of 22 even if his or her calculated MELD score is lower than that based upon his or her blood work. This criteria include patients with single lesions up to 5 cm, and <3 lesions ≤3 cm each. If a patient's MELD score is higher than 22 based upon his or her blood work then he or she would receive the higher score. Patients with hepatopulmonary syndrome and portopulmonary hypertension should be referred to a transplant center and may receive priority MELD points. Hepatopulmonary syndrome is described as hypoxemia and right to left shunting in patients with cirrhosis and portal hypertension. Shunting should be documented either by a positive contrast-enhanced transthoracic echocardiogram (bubble echo) or 99m Tc macroaggregated albumin study with greater than 6% brain uptake.[7]

Portopulmonary hypertension is a separate distinct entity that is associated with the development of vascular changes in the pulmonary bed indistinguishable from changes seen in patients with primary pulmonary hypertension. The diagnosis of portopulmonary hypertension requires the presence of portal hypertension and a mean pulmonary arterial pressure >25 mm Hg, pulmonary vascular resistance >120 dynes/cm^2, and pulmonary capillary wedge pressure <15 mm Hg.[7] Because both hepatopulmonary syndrome (HPS) and portopulmonary syndrome (PPH) may lead to progressive pulmonary hypertension that precludes liver transplantation, patients with either of these syndromes should be evaluated for liver transplantation before irreversible disease develops. Clinical signs of HPS or PPH are clubbing, low oxygen saturation, and shortness of breath out of proportion for what would be expected based on clinical exam or amount of ascites.

In some regions of the country, patients with hyponatremia receive MELD exception points. Patients with hyponatremia (serum sodium less than 130 mEq/L) have a 2-fold increased risk of death compared to patients with serum sodium greater than 130 mEq/L.[8]

MANAGEMENT OF COMPLICATIONS
AND ROUTINE FOLLOW-UP

Many patients think they are listed for liver transplant after their first visit to the transplant center despite education about the listing process and that it usually takes weeks to months to be listed for liver transplant depending on the circumstances. Transplant centers are required to notify patients when they are listed for liver transplant (and also if they are removed from the list) and should receive a letter stating so. It is good practice for the transplant center to send the referring physician a copy of the letter of listing as well.

Based on local practices, patients listed for liver transplant may be seen monthly to yearly at the transplant center depending on their severity of illness and MELD scores. For example, a patient with a MELD score of 12 listed for liver transplant may be seen every 6 to 12 months at the transplant center whereas a patient with a MELD score of 24 may be seen monthly. Much of the follow-up diagnostic testing for screening and surveillance of associated conditions can be arranged through the referring clinician's office. Transplant centers typically follow guidelines established by professional organizations, such as for screening or surveillance colonoscopy for polyps. Upper endoscopy to screen for esophageal varices may occur every 12 to 24 months.

Screening for hepatocellular carcinoma should occur every 6 months. Abdominal ultrasound is one method for screening and surveillance for HCC but in the United States there are limitations, using ultrasound to identify lesions in a cirrhotic liver. Cross-sectional imaging with CT or MRI is better at identifying small HCCs but CT is associated with radiation exposure and both are more expensive compared to ultrasound. A suggested surveillance schedule in patients listed for liver transplant is to alternate ultrasound with CT or MRI every 6 months. AFP is not recommended for screening for HCC because it has poor sensitivity, unless imaging is unavailable. Once a liver lesion suspicious for malignancy is identified in a cirrhotic liver, AFP should be obtained.

Management of Complications

Manifestations of end-stage liver disease include ascites, varices, and encephalopathy. Patients may live at a distance from the transplant center and it may not be practical to expect the patient to be followed for these complications at the transplant center. The referring clinician can usually manage these conditions and if additional expertise is needed, the patient can be referred to the transplant center.

Table 4-6

Suggested Management of Ascites

- Sodium restriction of less than 2 g daily
- Initiate therapy with spironolactone 50 mg daily
- If ascites poorly controlled, increase spironolactone 100 mg daily and furosemide 40 mg daily
- If ascites poorly controlled, check spot urine sodium/potassium ratio for compliance if less than 1 suggests noncompliance
- If compliant and ascites persists, continue to increase in 50-mg increments and furosemide in 20- to 40-mg increments until ascites is controlled or electrolyte disturbances occur
- If ascites remains poorly controlled and patient requires LVP every 1 to 2 weeks, consider TIPS

LVP, large-volume paracentesis; TIPS, transjugular intrahepatic portosystemic shunt.

Ascites

Ascites is the most common complication in patients with cirrhosis. Initial assessment includes a physical exam and imaging. Ascites may be a consequence of portal vein thrombosis and an assessment of the portal vein with an ultrasound with Dopplers should be obtained.

Initial treatment of ascites can be managed by the referring clinician and includes dietary restriction of sodium of less than 2 g daily. Fluid restriction should not be instituted unless the patient is hyponatremic. Spironolactone 50 mg daily may be prescribed for patients with mild to moderate ascites. Furosemide 40 mg daily can be added if ascites is not well controlled and spironolactone can be increased to 100 mg daily. The doses of spironolactone and furosemide can be increased sequentially usually keeping the 5:2 ratio until ascites is controlled or problems with hyperkalemia, hyponatremia, azotemia, or renal insufficiency develop. One approach is to tolerate a creatinine up to 1.5 to 2.0 mg/dL, a sodium of 128 mmol/dL, and potassium up to 5.5 mmol/dL. If gynecomastia or gynecomastalgia develops with spironolactone, it can be substituted with 5 to 10 mg of amiloride daily.

If ascites remains poorly controlled despite optimal doses of diuretics or electrolyte disturbances occur and the patient is requiring large volume paracentesis every 1 to 2 weeks, referral to the transplant center for a transjugular intrahepatic portosystemic shunt (TIPS) should be considered (Table 4-6). The transplant center may prefer to place the TIPS because of proper anatomical location in a potential liver transplant recipient. The TIPS should not be placed too proximally beyond the hepatic veins into the inferior vena cava (IVC) and not too distally beyond the extrahepatic portal vein or superior mesenteric vein. If the TIPS extends into the IVC or into the superior mesenteric vein (SMV) then the venous anastomoses at time of transplant may be very difficult or impossible.

TIPS is effective in reducing the need for large volume paracenteses (LVPs) and diuretic dose 75% of the time.[9] TIPS is associated with encephalopathy in up to 44% of patients, especially with the newer covered stents that are associated with lower rates of stenosis but higher rates of encephalopathy.[10] Thus, a patient who is on lactulose and rifaximin and has been hospitalized for encephalopathy may be a poor TIPS candidate. The portal vein needs to be patent; therefore, a patient with complete portal vein thrombosis or cavernous transformation may not be able to have a TIPS for technical reasons. Patients with advanced liver disease, such as those who have Child-Pugh class C cirrhosis, or patients with a MELD score greater than 18 are at risk from acute decompensation after TIPS and the transplant center should be involved in the decision to proceed with TIPS in these patients.

Patients with refractory ascites may best be managed with serial large volume paracenteses as needed. Patients who live far from their transplant center usually have ultrasound-guided paracentesis arranged through a local radiology department. Replacement with intravenous albumin is controversial although there is general agreement that patients without peripheral edema or with reduced glomerular filtration rates should receive 6 to 8 g of albumin per liter of ascites removed. This usually corresponds to 25 to 50 g of albumin (100 to 200 mL of 25% albumin solution) per paracentesis. Patients should have at least 1 serum albumin-ascitic fluid gradient (SAAG) determined to document ascites is from portal hypertension. A fluid cell count and culture should be ordered if spontaneous bacterial peritonitis is suspected.

Patients with a history of prior spontaneous bacterial peritonitis (SBP) should be placed on secondary prophylaxis. Daily prophylaxis with trimethoprim/sulfamethoxazole, ciprofloxacin, or norfloxacin is acceptable. Once weekly prophylaxis with ciprofloxacin is no longer recommended. Cirrhotic patients who present with SBP but do not have vomiting, hypotension, or significant electrolyte disturbances can be considered for outpatient therapy for SBP with an oral fluoroquinolone.

Primary prophylaxis for SBP in cirrhotic patients is controversial. The risk of the development of drug resistance needs to be weighed against the benefit of preventing infection. A randomized clinical trial of primary prophylaxis in patients with advanced cirrhosis demonstrated that patients with low protein ascitic level <15 g/L, Child-Pugh score >9, serum bilirubin >3 mg/dL, serum creatinine >1.2 mg/dL, blood urea nitrogen >25 mg/dL, or serum sodium <130 mEq/L demonstrated significantly lower rates of SBP and improved survival with norfloxacin prophylaxis. One year survival in the norfloxacin and placebo groups were 60% and 48%, respectively (p = 0.05).[11] It is reasonable to initiate primary prophylaxis in cirrhotic patients who meet these criteria.

Varices

Patients with cirrhosis should be screened for esophageal and gastric varices. Patients with grade 2 or greater esophageal varices or with gastric varices should be considered for prophylactic beta-blocker therapy. The goal is to reduce the risk of first variceal hemorrhage by reducing the resting heart rate by 25% or to approximately 60 beats per minute, but not at the expense of hypotension. Cirrhotic patients may have relative hypotension due to systemic vasodilatation and may not tolerate a blood pressure below 90/60 mm Hg. A reasonable starting dose is propranolol 20 mg oral twice a day or nadolol 40 mg daily. Primary prophylaxis with banding is usually reserved for patients who do not tolerate beta-blockers. A randomized clinical trial demonstrated more adverse events, chest pain, and bleeding with banding compared to beta-blockers.[12] On the other hand, beta-blockers may be associated with greater risk of hepatorenal syndrome in patients with ascites, and primary prophylaxis with banding may be appropriate in patients with ascites and large varices.

Esophagogastroduodenoscopy (EGD) with banding is effective as secondary prophylaxis for esophageal variceal bleeding and is used in conjunction with beta blockers. After initial esophageal variceal bleeding is stopped, repeat EGD with banding as needed should be scheduled every 2 to 4 weeks until varices are obliterated. Attempts at banding earlier may be met with large ulcers at the time of endoscopy. Proton pump inhibitors can be prescribed to decrease the size of banding ulcers. Once esophageal varices are obliterated, repeat endoscopy can be performed in 3 to 6 months and if no varices are banded, then annually.

When a cirrhotic patient presents with hematemesis and suspected variceal hemorrhage, there should be a low threshold to intubate the patient in order to secure the airway and optimize sedation. Although visualization may be difficult due to bleeding or reflux of blood into the esophagus, the esophago-gastric (EG) junction can usually be visualized and banding at the level of the EG junction should be performed if varices are present even if active bleeding is not seen. Continuous infusion of octreotide should be initiated and intravenous antibiotics, such as a fluoroquinolone or third-generation cephalosporin, should be prescribed to reduce the rate of bleeding and infection. There should be a low threshold to place a Minnesota or Blakemore tube if bleeding is uncontrollable and visualization is difficult. The gastric balloon should be inflated and pulled up against the EG junction. The esophageal balloon should almost never be inflated due to the risk of esophageal rupture.

The Minnesota tube can be placed through the mouth with an endoscope and snare at the end of the Minnesota tube to facilitate placement into the stomach. Verification of placement with an abdominal x-ray is advisable prior to inflation unless exsanguination is imminent. A randomized clinical trial demonstrated that proceeding directly to TIPS is associated with greater control of bleeding and a lower rebleeding rate compared to endoscopic therapy (97% versus 50%, p <0.001) and higher survival (86% versus 61%, p <0.001).[13] Thus, early TIPS for severe acute variceal bleeding should be considered.

Clinicians treating patients with end-stage liver disease often overlook malnutrition. A nutritional assessment with a dietician may be necessary in patients with signs of malnutrition to ensure adequate caloric intake and dietary supplementation with vitamins and minerals. Patients with cholestatic liver diseases may be deficient in the fat soluble vitamins (A, D, E, K) and alcoholic cirrhotics may develop deficiencies in vitamin B_{12}, thiamine, and folate. Nutritional supplements that have a high amount of calories and protein are frequently used to improve catabolism.

Encephalopathy

Changes in mental status are frequently due to portosystemic hepatic encephalopathy. The historic mainstay of treatment is lactulose to reduce colonic bacterial load that produces ammonia and to reduce the production of ammonia. The goal of treatment should be 2 to 4 bowel movements daily or less if symptoms are well controlled with less frequent bowel movements. The powder form of lactulose may be more palatable than the liquid form. Patients should not spend the entire day in the bathroom. If symptoms are not well controlled with lactulose, either neomycin 500 to 1000 mg 2 to 3 times a day or rifaximin 550 mg twice a day can be added. Rifaximin has been shown to reduce recurrent episodes of encephalopathy and hospitalizations by more than 50% compared to placebo and is now believed by many to be the drug of choice in combination with lactulose.[14] Ammonia levels are not useful for management, but instead history and clinical exam should guide management. Although encephalopathy may be debilitating, there is no standardized exception for liver transplantation for refractory encephalopathy.

Strategies for Increasing Organ Utilization

The disparity between the number of patients waiting for liver transplantation and the availability of deceased donor livers has led to the development of alternative transplant strategies to treat patients with end-stage liver disease (Table 4-7). The use of extended criteria donors (ECD) or segmental grafts (split deceased donor grafts or living donor liver transplant) are among some of the ongoing solutions. ECD or marginal donors describe donors or grafts that have characteristics associated with increased risk of graft

Table 4-7

Strategies for Increasing Utilization of Organs and Transplanting Patients

- Donation after cardiac death
- Hepatitis B core antibody donor livers for hepatitis B core and surface antibody positive recipients
- Hepatitis C donor livers for hepatitis C-positive recipients
- Split liver transplantation
- Adult to adult living donor liver transplantation

failure or donor-transmitted disease. A uniform definition of ECD has not been developed in liver transplantation, but many centers would consider older donor age, steatosis, donation after cardiac death (previously termed *non-heart beating donors*), hepatitis B core antibody donors, hepatitis C antibody-positive donors, hypernatremia, and prolonged cold ischemia time as factors associated with ECD.[15] However, liver transplantation has been performed with good outcomes from donors considered ECD, including transplanting livers from donors after cardiac death.[16]

The use of hepatitis B core antibody positive donors can be considered in candidates who are hepatitis B core antibody positive and hepatitis B surface antibody positive. The use of core antibody positive livers gives the candidate the possibility of receiving a liver transplant sooner than a candidate with a higher MELD score who is not hepatitis B core (IgG) and surface antibody positive. The risks and benefits of using a hepatitis B core antibody positive donor should be discussed with the patient and the patient should be formally consented if he or she agrees to accept a core antibody positive liver. The use of hepatitis B immune globulin and/or an oral nucleos(t)ide agent for prophylaxis against reactivation is variable among centers, although virtually all centers will prescribe some form of prophylaxis.

Adult Living Donor Liver Transplantation

Adult living donor liver transplantation (ALDLT) involves resecting the right lobe, left lobe, or left lobe with caudate lobe of a healthy person's liver and transplanting it to a suitable recipient after his or her cirrhotic liver is removed.[17] In ALDLT, both the donor and recipient need to be evaluated for surgery. The indications and evaluation of the ALDLT candidate are similar to the deceased donor candidate and the same contraindications apply. The potential benefit of ALDLT is to reduce waiting time mortality. However, the additional risk of morbidity and mortality to the donor needs to be considered. The risk of death to the donor is estimated to be 0.5%.[17] According to guidelines of the OPTN/UNOS Living Donor Committee, a team of clinicians should be assembled that evaluates the donor with at least one member who does not have a connection with the recipient's medical care or decision making.[18]

The optimal MELD score at the time of ALDLT may be in the range from 15 to 24, but this may vary on a case-by-case basis. Liver transplant candidates with MELD scores over 24 may require a whole liver in order to optimize their chance to survive the postoperative period. Patient and graft survival at 1 year were 89% and 81%, respectively, in recipients included in the National Institutes of Health (NIH) multicenter study of 9 centers that perform ALDLT (A2ALL consortium) and a survival benefit was demonstrated in those that proceeded to ALDLT rather than waiting on the list for potential deceased donor liver transplantation (DDLT).[19] The mean MELD score at the time of transplant was 15 + 6.9. Center experience is an important determinant of outcome with centers performing more than 20 ALDLTs having significantly lower risk of graft failure compared to less experienced centers.[19] Liver transplant candidates should be made aware of ALDLT as a potential option, especially in areas with long waiting times.

ECONOMICS OF LIVER TRANSPLANTATION

It is estimated that the charges associated with liver transplantation and the first year of care are $577,100.[20] The charges for a year of immunosuppressants are estimated at $23,300. Coverage of liver transplantation by health insurance is variable and out of pocket expenses for post-transplant medications can be significant. Most states' Medicaid plans cover the liver transplant procedure and the medications, including immunosuppression after the liver transplant. In contrast, patients on disability or who have Medicare may incur unaffordable expenses for post-transplant medications. The impact of the implementation of Medicare part D on liver transplant recipients has not been reported.

REFERENCES

1. Organ Procurement and Transplantation Network. Overall by organ: current U.S. waiting list. US Department of Health and Human Services. URL: http://optn.transplant.hrsa.gov/latestData/rptData.asp. Accessed July 5, 2012.

2. Wiesner R, Edwards E, Freeman R, et al. Model for end-stage liver disease (MELD) and allocation of donor livers. *Gastroenterology.* 2003;124(1):91-96.

3. Murray KF, Carithers RL Jr. AASLD practice guidelines: evaluation of the patient for liver transplantation. *Hepatology.* 2005;41(6):1407-1432.

4. Freeman RB Jr, Gish RG, Harper A, et al. Model for end-stage liver disease (MELD) exception guidelines: results and recommendations from the MELD exception study group and conference (MESSAGE) for the approval of patients who need liver transplantation with diseases not considered by the standard formula. *Liver Transpl.* 2006;12:S128-136.

5. Krahn LE, DiMartini A. Psychiatric and psychosocial aspects of liver transplantation. *Liver Transpl.* 2005;11(10):1157-1168.

6. Merion RM, Schaubel DE, Dykstra DM, Freeman RB, Port FK, Wolfe RA. The survival benefit of liver transplantation. *Am J Transplant.* 2005;5(2):307-313.

7. Krowka MJ. Hepatopulmonary syndrome and portopulmonary hypertension: implications for liver transplantation. *Clin Chest Med.* 2005;26(4):587-597.

8. Biggins SW, Kim WR, Terrault NA, et al. Evidence-based incorporation of serum sodium concentration into MELD. *Gastroenterology.* 2006;130(6):1652-1660.

9. Russo MW, Sood A, Jacobson IM, Brown RS Jr. Transjugular intrahepatic portosystemic shunt for refractory ascites: an analysis of the literature on efficacy, morbidity, and mortality. *Am J Gastroenterol.* 2003;98(11):2521-2527.

10. Riggio O, Angeloni S, Salvatori FM, et al. Incidence, natural history, and risk factors of hepatic encephalopathy after transjugular intrahepatic portosystemic shunt with polytetrafluoroethylene-covered stent grafts. *Am J Gastroenterol.* 2008;103(11):2738-2746.

11. Fernández J, Navasa M, Planas R, et al. Primary prophylaxis of spontaneous bacterial peritonitis delays hepatorenal syndrome and improves survival in cirrhosis. *Gastroenterology.* 2007;133(3):818-824.

12. Lo GH, Chen WC, Wang HM, Lee CC. Controlled trial of ligation plus nadolol versus nadolol alone for the prevention of first variceal bleeding. *Hepatology.* 2010;52(1):230-237.

13. Garíca-Pagán JC, Caca K, Bureau C, et al. Early use of TIPS in patients with cirrhosis and variceal bleeding. *N Engl J Med.* 2010;362(25):2370-2379.

14. Bass NM, Mullen KD, Sanyal A, et al. Rifaximin treatment in hepatic encephalopathy. *N Engl J Med.* 2010;362(12):1071-1081.

15. Feng S, Goodrich NP, Bragg-Gresham JL, et al. Characteristics associated with liver graft failure: the concept of donor risk index. *Am J Transplant.* 2006;6(4):783-790.

16. Tector AJ, Mangus RS, Chestovich P, et al. Use of extended criteria livers decreases wait time for liver transplantation without adversely impacting posttransplant survival. *Ann Surg.* 2006;244(3):439-450.

17. Russo MW, Brown RS Jr. Adult living donor liver transplant. *Am J Transplant.* 2004;4(4):458-465.

18. The Organ Procurement and Transplantation Network. Guidance for the medical evaluation of potential living donors. URL: optn.transplant.hrsa.gov/ContentDocuments/Guidance_MedicalEvaluationPotentialLivingLiverDonors.pdf. Accessed Sept 29, 2012.

19. Berg CL, Gillespie BW, Merion RM, et al. Improvement in survival associated with adult-to-adult living donor liver transplantation. *Gastroenterology.* 2007;133(6):1806-1813.

20. United Network for Organ Sharing. Costs. URL: http://www.transplantliving.org/before-the-transplant/financing-a-transplant/the-costs/. Accessed Sept 29, 2012.

5

Long-Term Management of the Liver Transplant Recipient

James F. Trotter, MD

The long-term management of the liver transplant recipient requires the diagnosis, evaluation, and treatment of a number of problems that can develop at any point after surgery. This chapter will summarize the basic principles of the more common problems that develop in clinical practice including immunosuppression, rejection, renal complications, recurrent disease, renal complications, evaluation of fever and diarrhea, biliary complications, infections, recurrent disease, malignancy, drug interactions, vaccinations, and bone disease.

Because of the success and widespread application of liver transplantation over the past 20 years, the number of transplant recipients continues to grow each year. Currently, there are more than 40,000 living liver recipients and their management requires knowledge in several specific areas of transplantation medicine. Post-transplant management begins immediately after the operation and the vigilance of monitoring varies based on the postsurgical interval. In the immediate postoperative period, the risk of complications is highest and their evolution can be rapid. Therefore, the patient is monitored on an hourly or daily basis until discharge, which usually occurs 1 to 3 weeks after surgery. In the outpatient setting, the patient is typically seen 2 to 3 times weekly for the first month and less frequently as time passes. Most transplant programs monitor laboratories at least every month during the

Brown RS Jr. *Common Liver Diseases and Transplantation: An Algorithmic Approach to Work-Up and Management (pp 65-78).*
© 2013 Taylor & Francis Group.

Table 5-1

Side Effect Profile of Common Immunosuppressants

	RENAL	HTN	DM	CHOL	GI	CYTOPENIA
Biologics						
Daclizumab	0	0	0	0	0	0
Basiliximab	0	0	0	0	0	0
Thymoglobulin	0	0	0	0	0	+
Alemtuzumab	0	0	0	0	0	+
Antimetabolites						
Azathioprine	0	0	0	0	++	++
Mycophenolates	0	0	0	0	++	++
Sirolimus	0	0	0	++	+	++
Calcineurin Inhibitors						
CSA	++	++	+	++	0	0/+
Tacrolimus	++	+	++	+	0	0/+
Steroids	0	++	++	++	0/+	0

0, none; +, less; ++, more.

HTN, hypertension; DM, diabetes mellitus; CHOL, hypercholesterolemia; GI, gastrointestinal symptoms; CSA, cyclosporine.

first year and then every month or every other month thereafter. Most programs mandate protocol follow-up clinic visits on a yearly basis to monitor for postoperative complications, especially in hepatitis C (HCV)-infected patients.

IMMUNOSUPPRESSION AND REJECTION

Most problems in liver recipients are either caused or aggravated by the chronic immunosuppression required to prevent rejection of the transplanted graft. The specific immunosuppressive regimen varies widely between transplant centers. However, the most common protocol is combination therapy of a calcineurin inhibitor (CNI), either tacrolimus or cyclosporine (CSA), along with an antimetabolite and corticosteroid (Table 5-1), most commonly tacrolimus (TAC) with mycophenolate mofetil (MMF) (or enteric-coated mycophenolic acid [MPA]) and a tapering dose of corticosteroids.[1] Tacrolimus is the most commonly administered immunosuppressant, prescribed to more than 90% of liver recipients. The side effects of TAC (and other immunosuppressants) are shown in Table 5-1, but the most common are renal toxicity, diabetes, and hypertension. The dose of CNIs is adjusted based on targeted trough blood levels (measured 12 hours after administration). Though doses and target levels vary by program and for each individual patient, a typical initial dose will be 4 to 10 mg daily in divided doses, with targeted blood levels of 8 to 12 ng/mL immediately after transplant when the highest level of immunosuppression is required. Thereafter, TAC levels are gradually tapered by 50% 1 year after transplant. MMF and MPA are administered at doses of approximately 1 to 2.0 g and 720 to 1440 mg divided twice daily, respectively, and blood levels are not monitored for either of these drugs. Approximately 50 % of liver recipients leave the hospital on MMF at the time of their transplant admission. Mycophenolate is most commonly used to allow a reduction in CNI levels to reduce nephrotoxicity associated with these drugs. Aside from gastrointestinal side effects (noted next), MMF causes thrombocytopenia or leukopenia which frequently limits its dosage to less than 2 g per day. The use of corticosteroids, once the mainstay of immunosuppression, has diminished in recent years due to their poor side effect profile and nontargeted immunosuppressive effects. In fact, about 25% of recipients are off the drug by the time of discharge and 50% by year 1. Other immunosuppressive agents are used less frequently and for specific indications. CSA, another CNI, is used less frequently instead of TAC. Sirolimus (SIR) is perhaps the most controversial immunosuppressant in that it has been the subject of multiple warnings against its use in liver transplantation by the FDA related to an increased risk of complications including graft loss and patient death. Despite these concerns, 10% of liver transplant recipients receive this drug during the first 2 years after transplant. SIR is administered once daily and the dose is adjusted based on targeted trough blood levels (measured 24 hours after administration) around 5 to 10 ng/mL. Similar to MMF, SIR is used primarily as a CNI-sparing agent to avoid renal toxicity. However, there are sparse data indicating that its administration mitigates this problem. SIR has an unusual side effect profile including an increased incidence of early hepatic artery thromboses in clinical trials, poor wound healing, hypercholesterolemia, cytopenia, and rarely pneumonitis. The poor wound healing and possible thrombotic risk has limited its use early post-orthotopic liver transplant and most programs use it after 1 month in patients with impaired renal function or prior malignancy. Azathioprine is infrequently used in liver transplantation and historically has been administered along with CSA. In addition, some clinicians find it particularly useful in the management of recurrent autoimmune hepatitis and as a substitute for MMF in women who are or might become pregnant. The final class of immunosuppressants is the biologic agents, antibodies to the T-cell, or one of its specific cellular receptors.[2] The immunosuppressive effects of the biologics are sustained days or weeks (or even months in the case of alemtuzumab) after their administration. However, they are poorly suited for chronic immunosuppression due to their parenteral administration and expense (as high as several thousand dollars per dose). Their primary advantage is the absence of renal toxicity. Therefore, biologics are used almost exclusively in the perioperative period when the recipient is vulnerable to acute renal failure or as treatment for severe rejection. In this setting, they may be used as the primary immunosuppressive agent in lieu of a CNI until renal function has improved. Finally, thymoglobulin and OKT3 are the biologic agents of choice for the treatment of steroid-resistant acute cellular rejection (ACR).

Rejection, categorized as acute or chronic, is perhaps the most important post-transplant complication, although the improved efficacy of the new immunosuppressive agents has decreased its occurrence to approximately 25%. Liver test abnormalities (elevated aspartate and alanine aminotransferase [AST and ALT, respectively]) are the first signs of acute cellular rejection (ACR) which explains the requirement for ongoing monitoring of liver function tests (LFTs) over the life of the patient. Once identified, LFT abnormalities require careful evaluation because manifestations of other common complications involving the liver graft (biliary, arterial, or infectious) may be similar. As a result, Doppler ultrasonography is required to exclude biliary dilatation, hepatic arterial occlusion, and hepatic abscess. In the absence of these findings, a liver biopsy is usually required to evaluate for the presence and severity of rejection and to exclude other problems such as cytomegalovirus, drug reaction, and others. The classic histologic features of ACR include endothelialitis, bile duct injury, and pancellular infiltrate including eosinophils. The severity of rejection may be graded using the Banff scale from 1 to 3 representing mild, 4 to 6 moderate, and 7 to 9 severe rejection. Treatment requires pulse doses of intravenous corticosteroids, although minor cases (Banff 1 to 3) may respond to an increase in the baseline immunosuppression. The precise treatment regimen for ACR varies by transplant center, but is typically 500 to 1000 mg methylprednisolone daily for 2 or 3 consecutive days. Response to treatment is usually rapid with a decrease in the AST by 50% or more (followed by ALT) within 1 to 2 days. In cases where the LFTs do not improve, a repeat liver biopsy is indicated to differentiate between steroid-resistant rejection and other causes of LFT elevation. Patients with steroid-resistant rejection require intravenous therapy with one of the potent biologic agents, usually OKT3 or thymoglobulin. The evaluation of elevated LFTs is a common and difficult management problem in patients with HCV. As discussed in detail on the next page, mild elevations in LFTs suggestive of ACR may also reflect histologic hepatitis due to recurrent viral infection, which is universal in HCV patients. In addition, the histologic distinction between ACR and recurrent HCV may be difficult. Chronic rejection is quite uncommon, but may occur in patients who are noncompliant with their immunosuppressive medication or who suffer recurrent bouts of ACR. As the name implies, its presentation is usually indolent over weeks to months and may be suspected in patients with a cholestatic pattern of LFT abnormalities (elevation in alkaline phosphatase [AP] and total bilirubin [TB]). The diagnosis is confirmed with liver biopsy where the histologic findings are minimal portal inflammation with bile duct injury or involution. Treatment is usually an increase in the baseline immunosuppression or addition of another immunosuppressant. The response to treatment is variable and some patients develop progressive graft failure leading to death or another transplant.

DRUG-DRUG INTERACTIONS

The potential for drug-drug interactions is particularly high in liver transplant recipients. While the list of interactions is innumerable, there are several common instances that require consideration. The most important interactions occur with the immunosuppressants metabolized through the hepatic cytochrome $P450_{3A4}$ system including TAC, CSA, and SIR. Patients receiving these medications who are prescribed another drug that may induce or inhibit P450 activity should either undergo careful monitoring to prevent high levels, which can lead to toxicity, or low levels, which can lead to rejection (Table 5-2). Alternatively, another noninteracting drug may usually be selected. The common clinical scenarios with P450 drug interactions include antibiotics/antifungals (azithromycin, ketoconazole, itraconazole, fluconazole) and antiseizure medications (phenytoin, carbamazepine). Another common instance where alterations in hepatic metabolism may alter drug levels is with HCV. Due to its effects on hepatic function, HCV infection decreases clearance of immunosuppressants cleared through the hepatic cytochrome P450 system. Therefore, in patients with severe recurrence of HCV where hepatic function is significantly impaired, marked elevations in blood levels will develop without a dose reduction. Conversely, patients experiencing viral clearance during interferon therapy for recurrent HCV may have significant improvement in hepatic function and therefore improved clearance of immunosuppressants. Such patients may require an increase in oral dosage to maintain adequate blood levels and adequate immunosuppression. Otherwise, graft rejection may develop.

Table 5-2

Cyclosporine/Tacrolimus Drug Interactions

DRUGS THAT INHIBIT CYTOCHROME P450 ENZYMES
Increase drug levels and lead to toxicity:
• Antifungals (fluconazole, itraconazole)
• Verapamil
• Erythromycin, clarithromycin, azithromycin
• Antihistamines
DRUGS THAT INDUCE CYTOCHROME P450 ENZYMES
Decrease drug levels and lead to rejection:
• Phenytoin
• Rifampin
• Barbiturates
• Alcohol

RENAL DISEASE

Renal disease occurs to some extent in almost all liver transplant recipients and the risk of developing renal failure is about 2% to 3% per year or 28% after 10 years.[3] The most common cause of renal failure is long-term exposure to CNIs along with the effects of diabetes and hypertension, which are further exacerbated by the CNIs. An additional problem is the growing proportion of liver candidates with renal disease due to inclusion of serum creatinine in the Model for End-Stage Liver Disease (MELD) score, which increases the transplant priority of with pre-existing renal injury.[4] There are 2 common strategies to prevent post-transplant renal disease, including a reduction in the dose and level of CNI to mitigate their nephrotoxic effects. Alternatively, the CNI may be discontinued altogether with replacement by MMF or SIR. Unfortunately, there is little evidence that either of these approaches reduces progressive renal failure. In some cases, liver transplant recipients with end-stage renal disease may undergo kidney transplantation after their liver transplant.

FEVER AND INFECTION

The evaluation of fever in the liver transplant recipient requires consideration of several possible diagnoses. As with any patient, the standard evaluation of chest radiograph, urinalysis, and blood cultures is indicated because urinary, respiratory, or blood infection is common. However, there are special considerations related to unusual infections that may occur more frequently in the liver recipient due to immunosuppression and complications in the hepatic graft. As noted below, cytomegalovirus (CMV) infection is common in the first few months after transplant, especially in patients who are CMV IgG negative receiving a graft from a CMV IgG positive donor. As compared to a bacterial infection, the fever pattern with CMV is more indolent, developing over several days and usually characterized by mild temperature elevation without temperature spikes. Fungal infections are uncommon despite immunosuppression and usually found in patients with multiple complications subjected to ongoing use of antibiotics. Cholangitis can occur due to a biliary obstruction and may be suspected if the patient has an elevated alkaline phosphatase and/or bilirubin. Unlike nontransplant patients, biliary obstruction may occur without bile duct dilatation. The diagnosis of a biliary obstruction may be suspected on ultrasound or MRCP and must be confirmed and treated with either endoscopic or percutaneous cholangiography. Hepatic or abdominal abscess is another consideration in the febrile liver recipient. This diagnosis can be difficult since symptoms may not be localized, especially with abdominal abscess. Therefore, the diagnosis of abdominal abscess should be considered in any patient with a persistent fever of unclear etiology. Finally, post-transplant lymphoproliferative disease (PTLD) may present as a fever as discussed next.

CYTOMEGALOVIRUS INFECTION

Due in large part to the requirement of immunosuppression, infections (bacterial, viral, fungal) are frequent in liver recipients. As in nonimmunosuppressed patients, bacterial infections are the most common, although liver recipients are at an increased risk for unusual infections due to the effects of chronic immunosuppression. CMV infection is a common problem particularly in patients who are "mismatched" (ie, those who have never been exposed to CMV [CMV IgG negative] receiving a liver from a donor with previous CMV exposure [IgG positive]).[5] Without proper prophylaxis, 80% of such liver recipients become viremic (CMV infection) and about one-half of those experience symptoms (CMV disease). CMV infection and disease usually occurs within 4 months of the transplant when immunosuppression is the highest and may present with indolent low-grade fevers, malaise, and cytopenia. Serious infections may develop as tissue invasive disease in the gastrointestinal tract, liver, or lungs. Therefore, mismatched patients, who are at the greatest risk for infection, should receive prophylaxis from the time of transplant surgery. Although the precise regimen varies between transplant centers, common protocols include oral ganciclovir, oral valganciclovir, or intermittent intravenous ganciclovir for approximately 8 weeks. With proper prophylaxis, the rate of CMV infection is reduced to less than 10%. Surveillance protocols to detect CMV viremia are utilized by some centers where blood virus levels are measured at prescribed post-transplant intervals (up to weekly). Pre-emptive therapy with ganciclovir or valganciclovir is initiated following detection of viremia to prevent the onset of symptoms. Another cohort of patients at risk for developing CMV infection are those receiving biologic agents (thymoglobulin or OKT3) for treatment of steroid-resistant rejection. In these cases, CMV prophylaxis is indicated.

DIARRHEA

Diarrhea is a common complication in the liver transplant recipient and is frequently due to an infection or medication side effect. Gastrointestinal symptoms, including diarrhea, are particularly common with MMF and a common reason for its discontinuation. Symptoms are usually evident within days or a few weeks after starting the drug. However, the occurrence of diarrhea may be less frequent with enteric-coated MPA, although there are little data to substantiate this claim. Tacrolimus is more frequently associated with diarrhea than the other CNI, CSA. Therefore, when diarrhea occurs in patients on MMF or TAC, a medication side effect should be considered. If possible, a dose reduction or change to another medication may help with the symptoms. Diarrhea can also represent a manifestation of CMV infection since gastrointestinal infection is common with this virus. In patients with primary sclerosing cholangitis (PSC), the occurrence of chronic ulcerative colitis may cause diarrhea after transplant even though the patient is receiving potent immunosuppressive therapy. Finally, *Clostridium difficile* colitis is common in liver transplant recipients and may be diagnosed initially with stool studies for the presence of white blood cells and/or specific tests for *C difficile*. Diarrhea may be treated empirically with metronidazole or medication adjustment. For persistent symptoms, a diagnostic flexible sigmoidoscopy or colonoscopy may be required to evaluate for infectious causes.

BILIARY COMPLICATIONS

Biliary complications are a frequent problem in liver transplant recipients and may manifest as LFT elevations (usually AP and TB), jaundice, right upper quadrant pain, or fever. Doppler ultrasonography is the most effective test to evaluate the patient with suspected biliary problems to identify biliary dilatation, hepatic abscess, biloma, as well as to exclude hepatic artery thrombosis, which is a common cause of biliary tract problems. Depending on the situation, direct visualization of the biliary tract via endoscopic retrograde cholangiography (ERCP) or percutaneous cholangiography (PTC) can provide diagnostic confirmation and potential treatment. PTC is used most often in patients whose biliary anastomosis (Roux-en-Y) is not easily amenable to ERCP. Patients with biliary strictures frequently respond to endoscopic stent placement along with antibiotic therapy. Clinicians frequently administer ursodeoxycholic acid to alleviate chronic complications of biliary strictures, primarily the formation of biliary sludge or stones. However, there is little evidence to support the benefit of this intervention. Biliary leaks may also be treated with stent placement, but depending on their nature and severity, they may require operative repair.

RECURRENT HEPATITIS C

Hepatitis C is the most common indication for transplant. Reinfection of the new graft is universal, so recurrent HCV is one of the most common and difficult postoperative management problems.[6] In fact, recurrent disease causes a 28% higher rate of graft loss compared to other patients. The diagnosis of recurrent HCV may be first suspected by a modest, but progressive LFT elevation usually occurring within weeks to months after the operation. However, in a small fraction (less than 5%), recurrence occurs immediately after surgery with marked aminotransferase elevations and jaundice. In this case, known as fibrosing cholestatic hepatitis (FCH), progressive graft failure and death usually occur in less than 1 year without antiviral treatment. A liver biopsy is indicated in all HCV patients with elevated LFTs. It determines the presence and severity of recurrent HCV and its differentiation from ACR. In addition, protocol yearly biopsies are indicated in all HCV patients to rule out progressive histologic disease in the absence of LFT abnormalities. The requirement for therapy (with pegylated interferon and ribavirin) is based on the severity of histologic findings.[7] Patients should be considered for treatment when stage 2 or higher fibrosis (on a scale of 0 to 4) is present on the biopsy or in any case of FCH. However, not all patients with the histologic requirement for therapy are suitable for interferon. The selection of patients for therapy must be balanced by the significant therapeutic side effects and limited efficacy with only 25% of patients experiencing sustained virologic response. Consequently, about 40% of patients are not eligible for therapy due to chronic medical problems which prohibit initiation of interferon therapy due to renal dysfunction, psychiatric problems, general debilitation, and cytopenias.

OTHER RECURRENT DISEASES

Besides HCV, other diseases may recur after transplant, although the consequences are typically less severe.[8] Hepatitis B (HBV), which accounts for only 5% of liver transplants, is rarely a problem after transplantation because of the highly effective prophylactic therapy.[9] The most commonly employed strategy to prevent HBV recurrence is parenteral administration of hepatitis B immune globulin (HBIg) (which binds and inactivates HBV surface antigen thereby preventing infection of the graft) along with oral antiviral therapy, typically entecavir and/or tenofovir. The dosing of HBIg varies between centers, but is initially up to 10,000 IU daily during the first postoperative week and then decreased progressively to once monthly. This protocol (of HBIg and oral antivirals) is over 90% effective in the prevention of recurrent HBV.[10] Because of the efficacy of the oral antiviral agents, many transplant centers have discontinued the long-term administration of HBIg.

Autoimmune hepatitis (AIH) recurs in many affected patients after transplant and often requires long-term administration of low-dose corticosteroid therapy to control. However, about 50% of patients with AIH may be managed effectively without corticosteroids. Despite recurrent disease, AIH rarely leads to graft loss as compared to HCV. Primary sclerosing cholangitis recurs in about 30% of patients, about one-half of whom develop progressive disease and require retransplantation. Treatment of post-transplant PSC recurrence is similar to before transplantation. Primary biliary cirrhosis (PBC) recurs in about 20% of patients but almost never leads to graft failure. As the occurrence of nonalcoholic steatohepatitis (NASH) increases, recurrence will likely become a problem. However, at this time, there are little to no data describing the frequency or severity of recurrent disease after transplantation. Alcoholic liver disease may also recur after transplantation. However, under the current selection process for transplantation, recurrence is uncommon and liver recipients whose underlying liver disease is from alcoholic cirrhosis have among the highest long-term survival rates of all patients.

MALIGNANCY AND POST-TRANSPLANT LYMPHOPROLIFERATIVE DISEASE

Malignancy is another disease that may occur more frequently in liver transplant recipients due to the effects of immunosuppression.[11] Chronic immunosuppression is thought to inhibit the natural surveillance immunity that is protective against neoplasia. In addition, many liver transplant recipients have an increased risk of cancer due to their underlying disease. The most common type of recurrent cancer after liver transplantation is hepatocellular carcinoma (HCC).[12] Approximately 25% of liver recipients have HCC at the time of transplant since carefully selected liver candidates with limited-stage (stage T2) disease receive a high priority for transplantation. In this population, the estimated risk of HCC recurrence after transplant is only 10%.[13] However, patients at the highest risk for recurrence are typically those who are understaged before transplant and discovered to have stage 3 or higher disease in their explant. In this situation, recurrence risk can be 50% or higher. Therefore, liver transplant recipients with HCC in the explant should be screened for recurrence after transplantation. The most commonly employed follow-up protocol is cross-sectional imaging and serum alpha-fetoprotein levels up to every 3 months during the first year and then up to yearly thereafter. Unfortunately, recurrent HCC is very difficult to treat and almost uniformly fatal. There is some evidence that specific immunosuppressives may provide some protection against recurrent HCC. In particular, the inhibitors of the mammalian target of rapamycin mTOR (SIR and everolimus) have potent in vitro antineoplastic properties. There are uncontrolled data demonstrating that these drugs may reduce HCC recurrence by as much as 50%. Another common post-transplant malignancy is PTLD, which is a unique form of lymphoma, occurring in about 1% of liver recipients. Patients at the greatest risk are those without exposure to Epstein-Barr virus (EBV) (IgG negative) who receive a liver from a donor who is EBV IgG positive. Since the risk of EBV acquisition increases with age, EBV mismatching is most likely to occur in pediatric liver recipients receiving grafts from adult donors. In these patients, some centers perform surveillance monitoring for EBV viremia and institute antiviral therapy with acyclovir to reduce the risk of PTLD. Similar to lymphoma, the presentation of PTLD is variable. Common symptoms include lymphadenopathy, fever, cytopenia, and weight loss. Unlike lymphoma, some cases of PTLD may be effectively treated without chemotherapy. In about one-half of the cases, the disease may be adequately controlled with a significant reduction or discontinuation of immunosuppression with or without antiviral therapy for EBV. Therefore, the first therapeutic maneuver following diagnosis is reduction of immunosuppression by 50%. In patients who are unresponsive or those with extensive disease, standard chemotherapy is indicated. One of the most commonly employed chemotherapeutics agents is the biologic agent rituximab, which is an antibody targeted against the CD-20 receptor on B lymphocytes.

Colon cancer is another common malignancy after liver transplantation particularly in patients with PSC and underlying chronic ulcerative colitis.[14] Such patients should undergo careful yearly screening with colonoscopy after transplantation. Finally, nasopharyngeal and pulmonary cancers are more frequent in recipients whose underlying disease is alcoholic cirrhosis. In these patients, the effects of cigarette smoking, which is very common in this population, are important risk factors. The most common form of cancer in liver transplant recipients is skin cancer, usually squamous cell carcinoma. Therefore, liver recipients should take particular caution toward reducing sun exposure through protective clothing and application of sunscreen and patients should have annual dermatologic evaluation. In addition, any suspicious lesions, especially in sun-exposed areas of the body, should be biopsied for the presence of skin cancer.

VACCINATION

Because of the increased risk of acquiring infectious diseases, careful observance of preventive vaccination protocols is essential for the liver transplant recipient. A comprehensive list of recommended vaccinations and their timing may be found through appropriate references.[15] Most patients will have received hepatitis A and B vaccinations during the pretransplant period. However, both are indicated in patients who have not been previously vaccinated in the absence of seroconversion to HAV IgG or HBV surface antibody, respectively. However, the efficacy rate for these vaccines is lower in immunosuppressed patients compared to the general population. In addition, vaccines for pneumococcus and influenza should be administered following routine guidelines. The use of live vaccines is contraindicated in all immunosuppressed patients including liver transplant recipients.

BONE DISEASE

Post-transplant osteoporosis is a particular problem, especially among women with cholestatic liver disease.[16] Many liver transplant candidates develop significant osteoporosis prior to transplantation and bone mineral density is further decreased during the first 3 months after surgery. Fracture rates as high as 30% have been reported in liver recipients with most fractures occurring within the first 2 years of transplantation. The cumulative steroid dose has been implicated in impairing bone formation and the trend toward decreasing their use may account for a slight reduction in post-transplant fracture rates over the past decade. Vitamin D levels should be checked on a regular basis and bone density performed at 1 year post-transplant and then every other year afterwards. Routine vitamin D and calcium supplementation is recommended at least while the patient is taking corticosteroids. Bisphosphonates can be used and are indicated for the prevention of steroid-induced bone loss. The treatment of post-transplant osteoporosis has become increasingly complex including calcium and vitamin D, as well as newer agents such as calcitonin and bisphosphonates.[17] Due to the complex nature of the diagnosis, management, and follow-up, treatment is best accomplished through specialty clinics.

SUMMARY AND KEY RECOMMENDATIONS

- The most common immunosuppressive therapy is tacrolimus with MMF and corticosteroids.
- Renal disease occurs to some extent in almost all liver transplant recipients and the risk of developing renal failure is about 2% to 3% per year or 28% after 10 years.
- Hepatitis C is the most common indication for transplant and reinfection of the new graft leads to recurrent disease and a 28% higher rate of graft loss compared to other patients.
- The most important drug interactions occur with the immunosuppressants metabolized through the hepatic cytochrome P450 system, including tacrolimus, CSA, and sirolimus.

REFERENCES

1. Fung J, Kelly D, Kadry Z, Patel-Tom K, Eghtesad B. Immunosuppression in liver transplantation: beyond calcineurin inhibitors. *Liver Transpl.* 2005;11(3):267-280.
2. Halloran PF. Immunosuppressive drugs for kidney transplantation. *N Engl J Med.* 2004; 351(26):2715-2729.
3. Ojo AO, Held PJ, Port FK, et al. Chronic renal failure after transplantation of a nonrenal organ. *N Engl J Med.* 2003;349(10):931-940.
4. Charlton MR, Wall WJ, Ojo AO, et al. Report of the first international liver transplantation society expert panel consensus conference on renal insufficiency in liver transplantation. *Liver Transpl.* 2009;15(11):S1-34.
5. Razonable RR. Cytomegalovirus infection after liver transplantation: current concepts and challenges. *World J Gastroenterol.* 2008;14(31):4849-4860.

6. Terrault NA. Hepatitis C therapy before and after liver transplantation. *Liver Transpl.* 2008;14(suppl 2):S58-66.

7. Watt K, Veldt B, Charlton M. A practical guide to the management of HCV infection following liver transplantation. *Am J Transplant.* 2009;9(8):1707-1713.

8. O'Grady JG. Phenotypic expression of recurrent disease after liver transplantation. *Am J Transplant.* 2010;10(5):1149-1154.

9. Samuel D. The option of liver transplantation for hepatitis B: where are we? *Dig Liver Dis.* 2009;41(suppl 2):S185-189.

10. Coffin CS, Terrault NA. Management of hepatitis B in liver transplant recipients. *J Viral Hepat.* 2007;14(suppl 1):37-44.

11. Watt KD, Pedersen RA, Kremers WK, Heimbach JK, Sanchez W, Gores GJ. Long-term probability of and mortality from de novo malignancy after liver transplantation. *Gastroenterology.* 2009;137(6):2010-2017.

12. Yao FY. Liver transplantation for hepatocellular carcinoma: beyond the Milan criteria. *Am J Transpl.* 2008;8(10):1982-1989.

13. El-Serag HB, Marrero JA, Rudolph L, Reddy KR. Diagnosis and treatment of hepatocellular carcinoma. *Gastroenterology.* 2008;134(6):1752-1763.

14. Trotter JF. Cancer surveillance following orthotopic liver transplantation. *Gastrointest Endosc Clin N Am.* 2001;11:199-214.

15. Vaccines and immunizations: recommendations and guidelines. URL: http://www.cdc.gov/vaccines/recs/default.htm. Centers for Disease Control Prevention, Department of Health and Human Services. Accessed February 1, 2011.

16. Stein E, Ebeling P, Shane E. Post-transplantation osteoporosis. *Endocrinol Metab Clin North Am.* 2007;36(4):937-963.

17. Collier J. Bone disorders in chronic liver disease. *Hepatology.* 2007;46(4):1271-1278.

6

Hepatitis B Virus

Blaire E. Burman, MD and Robert S. Brown Jr, MD, MPH

Hepatitis B is the most prevalent liver disease worldwide. More than 2 billion individuals have been infected with HBV and an estimated 350 to 400 million people are living with chronic infection, as identified by the persistence of hepatitis B surface antigen (HBsAg) positivity after initial exposure.[1] Each year over 1.2 million deaths are attributable to the consequences of hepatitis B: cirrhosis, liver failure, and hepatocellular carcinoma (HCC). In the United States, considered a low-prevalence country, nearly 1.4 million are known to have chronic hepatitis B (CHB) yet it is estimated that the majority of patients infected are undiagnosed due to lack of public awareness, inadequate screening, and access to medical services.[2-4] More than 1 in 4 of those infected early in life will go on to develop liver cancer or cirrhosis.[5] With continued adherence to vaccination and case prevention, improved screening, disease monitoring, and treatment of appropriate candidates, these complications are preventable. CHB remains a significant public health problem despite advances in our understanding of the natural history of disease, availability of more sensitive diagnostic tests, and access to more effective antiviral therapies.

The worldwide prevalence of infection is distributed widely yet unequally, with a higher burden of disease within certain geographic regions, namely Asia, sub-Saharan Africa, the Pacific Islands, Eastern Europe, and among

Brown RS Jr. *Common Liver Diseases and Transplantation:*
An Algorithmic Approach to Work-Up and Management (pp 79-97).
© 2013 Taylor & Francis Group.

particular subpopulations with behavioral risk factors. Approximately 45% of the world's population lives in areas of high endemicity, where the prevalence of CHB is >8%. In the United States, pockets of high prevalence are found in communities of immigrants born in endemic countries.[6] Over the past 2 decades, the incidence of acute HBV infection has decreased dramatically in the United States and around the world, attributable to the advent of an effective vaccination and uptake of universal neonatal immunization campaigns. However, a significant burden of established disease exists in the United States. Prevalence remains high among immigrant communities and those with behavioral risk factors, a majority of whom are not well-integrated into health care and are not appropriately screened. Hence, the majority of CHB in the United States is undiagnosed or untreated. Hepatitis B is both preventable and treatable, yet morbidity and mortality attributable to chronic HBV remains inadequately addressed.

Although the treatment of CHB with interferon or oral antiviral therapy usually occurs in a specialist gastroenterology or hepatology clinic, it is critical that all health care professionals be adept in appropriate screening and case identification, initial evaluation, and monitoring of chronic disease. It is estimated that only a fraction of patients who would benefit from antiviral therapy ever receive such treatment.[3] The natural history of CHB is highly variable and dependent on host, viral, and environmental factors that dictate viral replication and immune response. While the majority of patients will remain asymptomatic, recurrent bouts of immune activity and resultant hepatocellular inflammation can lead to fibrosis and progress to end-stage liver disease. Furthermore, the HBV integrates into host hepatocytes and acts as a reservoir of persistent infection and precursor of liver cancer.[7] The goal of antiviral therapy is not to cure hepatitis B but to suppress viral replication and prevent ongoing immune activity. There are effective therapeutic options but some controversy remains over the optimal time to initiate and duration of treatment. A set of algorithms have been developed to help health care professionals effectively identify cases of CHB, monitor disease activity, and refer for treatment when appropriate.

POPULATIONS AT RISK: WHO TO SCREEN

An effective vaccination against hepatitis B has been widely available and since 1991, recommended by the World Health Organization (WHO) for all neonates and catch-up vaccinations for older age groups in areas with HBV prevalence rates above 2% or high-risk behavioral groups.[8] This approach has significantly decreased rates of incident infection, yet does not address the growing reservoir of existing carriers. In order to eliminate HBV transmission in the United States and decrease HBV-related morbidity and mortality, people with chronic HBV infection must be identified and monitored. Carriers of HBV are often asymptomatic, unaware of their infection, and thus have the potential for transmitting the virus to others or developing severe liver disease later in life. In order to interrupt ongoing transmission, it is essential to screen high-risk populations, now more broadly defined, in order to identify and vaccinate susceptible contacts and prevent vertical transmission. Furthermore, all people with chronic HBV require close medical management to identify progression of liver disease, manage complications, and initiate antiviral therapy.

All people in high-risk groups and patients with elevated liver enzymes or evidence of active liver disease without an identified cause should be screened. The global distribution of hepatitis B infection is highly variable; countries are defined as having high, intermediate, or low prevalence based on the estimated prevalence of HBsAg carriers of greater than 8%, between 2% and 7%, or less than 2%, respectively (Table 6-1). Nearly half of the world population lives in regions in which HBV is highly endemic.[9] Prevalence is generally low in more developed countries and the majority of cases are identified in people immigrated from high or intermediate prevalence countries and those with behavioral risk factors. The CDC previously recommended HBsAg testing for people born in countries with greater than 8% prevalence, all pregnant women, infants born to HBsAg-positive mothers, close contacts of HBV-infected people, and those with known acute exposure who may benefit from postexposure prophylaxis.[10] A 2008 report updated these guidelines to include people born in countries with HBsAg prevalence over 2% and those with behavioral risk factors, namely injection drug users, and men who have sex with men. These established high-risk groups should be screened for HBV infection and immunized if HBsAg seronegative.[6,11,12]

Routine screening tests should include a serologic assay for HBsAg and antibodies to hepatitis B surface and core antigens (ie, HBsAb, HBcAb). A confirmed HBsAg-positive test is indicative of active infection, either acute or chronic, and chronic infection can be confirmed by the absence of IgM anti-HBc or by the persistence of HBsAg or HBV DNA viral load for greater than 6 months (Table 6-2). Positive results should be accompanied by appropriate clinical evaluation, counseling, and referral for further care. For people who are at ongoing risk for infection, a negative HBsAb test indicates lack of immunity and these patients should be vaccinated. A subgroup of people may test positive for isolated anti-HBc, but not for HbsAg or surface antibodies. This may occur in a number of settings, primarily immunity after recovering from a prior infection, but also the window phase of acute hepatitis B, and when serum HbsAg levels have decreased to undetectable levels despite active HBV viral replication within hepatocytes (Table 6-3).[13,14]

Table 6-1

High-Risk Groups: Who to Screen

PEOPLE BORN IN AREAS OF HIGH OR INTERMEDIATE PREVALENCE FOR HBV
• Asian-Pacific region
• Middle East
• European-Mediterranean region, including Greece, Italy, Portugal, Spain, and Malta
• Eastern Europe
• South America
• Caribbean region
• Native populations of the Arctic
OTHER HIGH-RISK GROUPS
• Household and sexual contacts of HBsAg+ people
• People with history of IV drug use
• People with multiple sexual partners or personal history of STDs
• Men who have sex with men
• Correctional facility inmates
• People with chronic elevation of ALT or AST
• People with HIV or HCV
• Patients undergoing renal dialysis
• All pregnant women

NATURAL HISTORY

HBV is transmitted through infected blood or body fluids via percutaneous, sexual, or perinatal exposure, in addition to close contact between people, especially children, in hyperendemic areas. Primary HBV infection is most commonly asymptomatic. Infected patients will either clear the virus from the bloodstream and liver and go on to develop prolonged immunity to reinfection or enter a state of chronic infection with ongoing viral replication. Unique to this virus, the risk of progression from acute to chronic HBV infection is inversely related to the patient's age and influenced by immune status at acquisition. Further, the cumulative rate of morbidity and mortality related

Table 6-2

Serologic Features of Hepatitis B Virus Infection

	ACUTE HBV	RECOVERY FROM ACUTE HBV	CHRONIC HBV	CHRONIC HBeAg NEGATIVE HBV	INACTIVE CARRIER STATE
HBsAg	X (may clear)		X	X	X
Anti-HBsAb		X			
Anti-HBc	X	X	X	X	X
Anti-HBc IgM	X				
HBeAg	X		X		
Anti-HBeAb		X (in some cases)		X	X

Table 6-3

Screening Algorithm for Patients at Risk for Hepatitis B Virus

Screen for HBsAg, HBsAb, and HBcAb, then:
- If positive, then further testing: HBeAg, HBeAb, HBV DNA viral load
- If negative, then vaccinate

to CHB is highest among those who acquire infection as neonates or in early childhood. Hence, those infected early in life are most likely to develop lifelong infection and suffer clinical consequences from HBV. Once chronic infection is established, the natural course of disease is a dynamic interplay of viral and immune factors.

In hyperendemic areas where HBV infection is acquired during childbirth, there is a high level of immunologic tolerance and in greater than 90% of newborns chronic lifelong infection ensues. Children infected between the ages of 1 and 5 have an intermediate 50% risk of developing chronic infection. In contrast, most infections in low prevalence regions occur during adolescence and early adulthood through behavioral exposures, such as sexual or close personal contact. In immune competent adults, a strong cellular immune response invokes clinically apparent acute hepatitis, but a vast majority clear the virus, such that less than 5% of healthy adults develop CHB.[13] People with suppressed immunity (ie, HIV positive, patients on chemotherapy or systemic steroids) are less likely to clear infection at any age and a higher proportion will progress to chronic disease once exposed. These patients are also at risk for reactivation of previously cleared hepatitis B.

After primary infection occurs, there is an incubation period of 4 to 10 weeks before HBsAg becomes detectable in the peripheral blood. At this time, viremia is well established and viral titers are high during acute infection. Shortly thereafter, anti-HB core IgM antibodies develop. In a majority of cases, HBeAg is detectable, and the continued presence of this marker is indicative of high titers of HBV in the blood, typically at levels of 100,000 IU/mL or higher.[15] Infection is cleared from hepatoctyes without clinically significant immune activation in most cases and the viral antigens HBsAg and HBeAg are purged from circulation. IgM is detectable for the first 6 months, then anti-HBc IgG persists indefinitely as a marker of past infection rather than vaccination. Antibodies against HBsAg signify recovery from acute infection and protective immunity from reinfection. Complete eradication of HBV infection is the exception to the rule, however, as stable HBV DNA becomes integrated into the host genome and so-called "inactive" infection is established in the majority of those infected.

Ongoing HBV replication is the most significant risk factor for progression of chronic infection to clinical disease. The relationship between HBV DNA levels and the development of liver injury was established by the REVEAL study, a large prospective cohort study that showed the cumulative incidence of cirrhosis and HCC increased linearly with DNA levels.[16] Patients with increasing levels over time or with persistently elevated levels at follow-up were at the highest risk. The data were reanalyzed after more sensitive PCR assays for DNA quantification were introduced, and revealed that risk was most significant with HBV DNA levels greater than 10^6 copies, which inform current treatment guidelines. Surprisingly, development of cirrhosis was independent of serum ALT and HBeAg status in this study, although ALT normalization and HBeAg seroconversion remain important goals of therapy.[16-18] Overall, a complex interplay of viral, immune, and environmental factors influence disease severity and progression and render CHB a challenging condition to monitor and manage.

PHASES OF CHRONIC INFECTION

Chronic HBV can be divided into 4 dynamic yet distinct phases that correlate with the host immune response and are characterized by distinct serologic and inflammatory markers: immune active, immune tolerant, inactive chronic carrier state, and reactivation. Progression through these phases is nonlinear and not all patients will experience each phase of infection. Generally, HBV acquisition in early childhood is followed by immune tolerance for a number of years, often 2 to 3 decades. In contrast, acquisition later in life is followed by a very short, if any, period of immune tolerance.

Transition to the immune active or clearance phase is heralded by high HBV DNA levels with fluctuating levels of ALT, which correspond to ongoing or intermitted hepatic inflammation and variable progression toward fibrosis or cirrhosis. For some patients, the immune active phase can lead to spontaneous HBeAg seroconversion with loss of HBeAg and development of anti-HBe antibodies. Other patients may seroconvert with antiviral therapy ,which helps the immune system clear the virus from the blood stream by suppressing viral replication. Alternatively, patients may relapse from inactive CHB to a reactivation phase, either spontaneously or by virtue of HBV therapy withdrawal or immune suppression. An additional group of patients in the reactivation phase have HBeAg-negative CHB associated with precore and/or double-base care promoter mutant virus.

The *immune tolerance* phase is characterized by normal transaminase levels and minimal histologic changes despite high HBV DNA titers with wild-type, HBeAg-positive virus. Treatment is not efficacious in this phase and patients should be monitored with ALT testing every 3 to 6 months. Given that ALT levels tend to fluctuate and may be elevated from causes other than viral hepatitis, liver biopsy can be helpful to identify the subset of patients with significant inflammation or fibrosis who may benefit from therapy. At some point, most patients in the immune tolerant phase will mount an enhanced immune response and transition to the immune active phase. This transition most commonly occurs between the ages of 20 and 40 in patients who acquired HBV infection perinatally, earlier for those who were infected in childhood, and can be immediate for those with primary acquisition in adulthood.[19]

The *immune active* phase is marked by high levels of DNA in addition to ALT elevations and evidence of inflammation on liver biopsy as the body tries to clear wild-type virus. Periods of disease activity during which serum ALT is raised represent the major opportunity for effective treatment. Patients with persistent immune active chronic infection should therefore be on antiviral therapy to prevent progressive liver fibrosis, particularly if moderate to severe hepatitis is apparent on biopsy. Patients in the immune active phase are typically HBeAg positive and can spontaneously clear HBeAg and develop anti-HBe antibodies at a rate of 5% to 15% per year, while others may seroconvert on effective therapy.[20] Although we now know that a subset of HBeAg-negative patients have active viral replication, seroconversion is often used as an endpoint of therapy and a marker of less active disease. Patients who remain in the immune active phase for years typically develop progressive liver fibrosis and harbor a greatly elevated risk for clinically significant cirrhosis and hepatocellular carcinoma.

The majority of patients with CHB will eventually enter an *inactive carrier state* marked by clearance of wild-type HBeAg-positive virus, generation of anti-HBe antibodies, normalization of ALT, and resolution of hepatic inflammation. HBV DNA is still present in the serum but at lower levels. Approximately one-half of patients infected in adulthood will enter this phase within 5 years of infection, and a majority within a decade. Of patients who persist in the inactive carrier state, the majority will remain HBeAg-negative and can be monitored less frequently. However, between 20% and 30% will experience a *reactivation phase* of immune active disease after years of inactivity.[20] This can be spontaneous or secondary to immunosuppressive or cytotoxic chemotherapy, which leads to reactivation of active infection and viral replication in 20% to 50% of patients.[21] Alternatively, a small minority of patients in the inactive carrier state, approximately 0.5% to 1%, will lose HBs antigen entirely over time.[22] This is attributed in part to the compartmentalization of closed circular DNA within hepatocytes, which serve as latent viral reservoirs that are not detectable in peripheral blood. Clearance of HBsAg therefore does not always signify resolution of infection and even HBsAg-negative patients, usually who are HBcAb-positive, can undergo reactivation.

It was previously assumed that HBeAg seronegativity was associated with lower levels of circulating HBV DNA and the development of an inactive carrier state. It is now known that approximately one-third of HBeAg-negative carriers enter a reactivation phase and experience either intermittent or persistent immune activity with ALT flares and may in fact have high levels of viremia. This state, clinically termed *HBeAg-negative CHB* is associated with the presence of precore and/or double base core promoter mutations, which downregulate or prevent the production of e antigen. Since HBeAg seroconversion has been an important endpoint for therapy, the most appropriate clinical management strategy and on-therapy monitoring for these patients is controversial. Most HBeAg-negative patients have genotype C or D virus and are from southern Europe or Asia, but the prevalence has increased worldwide. Treatment of patients with HBeAg-negative hepatitis has been discouraging; only 15% to 27% have sustained virologic responses to standard interferon, and although antiviral agents can suppress the virus and lead to undetectable HBV DNA levels, indefinite treatment is required.[5]

Table 6-4

Pretreatment Evaluation

HISTORY AND PHYSICAL
• Risk factors for viral hepatitis and route of transmission
• Likely duration of infection
• Risk factors for HIV/HCV coinfection
• Alcohol history
• Comorbid diseases
• Family history of HCC
PRETREATMENT TESTS
• Serial testing of ALT and HBV DNA levels
• Liver function tests
• HBeAg and anti-HBeAb
• HBV genotype
• Full viral hepatitis panel and HIV testing
• HCC screening in high risk patients
• Liver biopsy in select patients

PRINCIPLES OF TREATMENT

Hepatitis B can be clinically silent for many years, yet eventually have a significant impact on morbidity and survival. All patients with CHB should be considered for therapy and receive comprehensive pretreatment evaluation (Table 6-4). Primary goals of treatment include suppression of viral replication, interruption of necroinflammatory injury, and prevention of clinical progression to cirrhosis, liver failure, and liver cancer. Patients in the immune active or reactivation phases clearly benefit from antiviral therapy, but given the dynamic nature of HBV infection the decision of whom to treat and at what stage is not always straightforward. Patients without clinical evidence of disease require close monitoring. Rising levels of ALT and/or serum HBV DNA indicate immune activity that, if left unchecked, will likely progress to fibrosis. Certain host factors including genotype, gender, age of acquisition, coinfection with HCV or HIV, and immune suppression favor starting therapy given the higher risk of complications. Close monitoring is key not only in monitoring efficacy and delineating treatment duration, but in

---

Box 6-1

When to Refer

While the majority of patients with CHB can be managed by primary care physicians, treatment of certain high risk groups should be guided by a hepatology specialist. This includes patients with end-stage liver disease, those listed for or following liver transplantation, HBsAg-positive patients undergoing immunosuppressive or cancer chemotherapy, patients with viral coinfections, and pregnant women with high viral load or immune active disease.

---

identifying the emergence of virologic breakthrough and drug resistance as well.

According to updated guidelines, treatment is indicated for all patients with clinically decompensated HBV cirrhosis, HBeAg-positive patients with serum HBV DNA above 20,000 IU/mL, HBeAg-negative patients with HBV DNA above 2,000 IU/mL, and patients with ALT levels greater than twice the upper limit of normal regardless of serostatus.[5] It is important to note, however, that DNA levels fluctuate and a significant number of patients progress to clinical disease despite DNA levels below threshold. In fact, approximately 15% of patients with HCC related to hepatitis B have serum DNA levels of less than 2,000 IU/mL.[18] Further, there is not always a direct correlation between the degree of increase in ALT and the extent of necroinflammatory activity in the liver. Up to one-third of patients with persistently normal ALT levels will have evidence of fibrosis on biopsy, particularly older patients and those with pre-existing cirrhosis. Hence, liver biopsy becomes important for patients who do not meet all above criteria; patients with ALT between 1 to 2 times the upper limit of normal and HBV DNA between 2000 and 20,000 IU/mL should be considered for treatment if biopsy reveals moderate to severe hepatitis or significant portal fibrosis. Hence, both viral and host factors for disease progression need to be considered in the decision to initiate therapy (Box 6-1).

THERAPEUTIC OPTIONS

The decision to initiate treatment or to monitor disease activity without active therapy must be made on a case-by-case basis. Deciding which agent to use should also be individualized. Despite an increasing armament of licensed drugs for the treatment of CHB, long-term efficacy is limited by poor tolerability particularly of interferon, low sustained "off therapy" viral response, and the development of viral resistance to oral antivirals. Eradication of HBV continues to be a rarely achieved goal in clinical practice and the overarching aim of therapy is to prolong suppression of viral replications and prevent complications of chronic infection while minimizing the burden of drug side effects and antiviral resistance. Effective therapy can, however, prevent progression to clinical liver disease and greatly diminish the risk of hepatocellular carcinoma. There are currently 7 licensed agents for the treatment of hepatitis B, including 2 immunomodulators (interferon alfa-2b, peginterferon alfa-2a) and 5 nucleos(t)ide analogs (lamivudine, adefovir, entacavir, tenofovir, telbivudine), which may be used as monotherapy or in combination. Each category has unique benefits and disadvantages but at present, preferred first-line treatment choices are entecavir, tenofovir, and peginterferon alfa-2a based on superior efficacy and tolerability in clinical trials. It is important to note that existing therapies can effectively manage nearly 95% of chronic infections, but the majority of cases remain undiagnosed and untreated.[23]

Interferon alfa-2a (IFN) therapy has nonspecific antiviral, antiproliferative, and immunomodulatory effects. Pegylated IFN has largely replaced standard IFN in clinical practice due to improved activity, convenience, and side effect profile. IFN has proven most effective in patients with HBeAg-positive disease, active viral replication, and elevated ALT suggestive of active hepatic inflammation and better outcomes with genotype A HBV. Treatment is given in a defined and self-limited course, usually 48 weeks, and is not associated with the development of drug resistance so future treatment options with oral antivirals are preserved. IFN is limited, however, by numerous contraindications to starting therapy and side effects on therapy, including flu-like symptoms, nausea, headache, and psychological disturbances, which often lead to treatment discontinuation. In general, IFN therapy is best suited for young patients with well-compensated HBeAg-positive CHB. While most will not achieve a negative viral load, one-third of patients with HBeAg-positive infection experience HBeAg seroconversion, which is a durable response after treatment withdrawal for up to 90% of patients[24] IFN can lead to intermittent ALT "flares" in up to half of patients, which, while unsettling, may indicate immune-mediated clearance and a favorable response. There is controversy, however, about the safety of IFN in patients with cirrhosis who are at risk for clinical decompensation with hepatitis flares. Overall, the need for frequent injections and multiple side effects makes patients with CHB less likely to choose interferon as a first-line treatment.

Direct oral antiviral agents are more potent inhibitors of viral replication and achieve initial "on-therapy" responses in the majority of patients, and are therefore more appropriate for patients with active viral replication and high HBV DNA levels. However, long-term therapy is required for sustained efficacy given that reactivation following discontinuation of treatment is the rule. For those patients with decompensated cirrhosis, lifelong therapy and consideration for transplant is necessary. Of the 5 oral agents now available, first line use of adefovir, telbivudine, and lamivudine has fallen out of favor. Lamivudine was once the first-line oral agent but is associated with high rates of drug resistance and is rarely initiated in treatment-naïve patients but may be continued in those with sustained response. Telbivudine is a more potent agent but also has a low barrier to resistance and exhibits crossresistance with lamivudine. Adefovir has relatively low rates of resistance but has intermediate antiviral activity with lower rates of viral suppression, ALT normalization, and histologic improvement than the first-line oral agents entecavir and tenofovir.[5]

Pegylated interferon alfa-2a, tenofovir, and entecavir have been identified as first-line therapy for treatment-naïve patients based on recent clinical trials. Entecavir is the most potent available agent but can be less effective in patients who already carry lamivudine mutations. Tenofovir is the most recently approved agent and has performed well in superiority trials, but does require dose adjustment for renal failure, and monitoring of creatinine and phosphorus is recommended given reports of renal insufficiency and osteomalacia. For patients who have been successfully treated with a second-line antiviral, there is no need to switch agents if serum HBV DNA levels remain persistently low or undetectable. Data on the efficacy of de novo combination therapy are limited but initial studies did not demonstrate a synergistic effect or additional clinical benefit with regard to traditional endpoints for either interferon plus antiviral or dual antiviral therapy regimens. On the other hand, the addition of a second antiviral to a failing monotherapy course is preferable to switching agents in terms of minimizing further multi-agent resistance. For example, the addition of adefovir to the regimen of patients who develop on-treatment lamivudine resistance can prevent virologic and clinical breakthroughs and has better outcomes than discontinuing lamivudine.[25]

Monitoring Response to Therapy

Patients should be monitored carefully during treatment with serum ALT and HBV DNA every 3 to 6 months to determine therapeutic efficacy (Table 6-5). Favorable response to antiviral therapy can be heralded by normalization of ALT, a decrease in serum HBV DNA level, loss of HBeAg, and improvement in liver histology. Over time, it appears possible to reverse fibrosis and even early cirrhosis with effective therapy. An initial response is typically measured at 12 to 24 weeks and, if achieved, the goal is to maintain on-therapy suppression. While CHB is not considered curable, the ultimate aim of treatment is to achieve sustained off-therapy response with

Table 6-5

Treatment Response

RESPONSE TO ANTIVIRAL THERAPY	DEFINITION
Primary treatment failure	HBV DNA is not reduced by at least 1 log10 IU/mL at week 12
Inadequate virologic response	HBV DNA remains >2000 IU/mL at week 24
Partial virologic response	HBV DNA is <2000 but still detectable at week 24
Complete virologic response	HBV DNA undetectable at week 24; can be sustained on-therapy or off-therapy
Virologic breakthrough	Increase in serum HBV DNA level by >1 log10 IU/ mL above nadir after initial virologic response achieved on therapy
Biochemical breakthrough	Increase in ALT level above upper limit of normal after achieving normalization on therapy

maintenance of biochemical and virologic suppression after drug discontinuation. Given that reactivation of viral replication is an omnipresent risk, the appropriate time to stop treatment and whether to stop at all is a subject of debate.

The longer active viral replication continues unchecked despite antiviral therapy, the greater the chance for virologic and biochemical breakthrough and the development of resistance. Primary treatment failure is defined as failure to reduce serum HBV DNA by 1 log10 IU/mL at week 12 in a patient with strict adherence and should prompt a switch to more potent or combination therapy. Inadequate or partial virologic response is defined by residual HBV DNA at week 24 and can be managed either by continuing current therapy, switching agents, or adding an additional agent with a different resistance profile.

Antiviral Resistance

The primary limitation of prolonged oral antiviral therapy is the development of drug resistance, though this risk is greatly diminished with newer agents. Initial signs of resistance include rebound of HBV DNA levels (virologic breakthrough), subsequent rise in ALT (biochemical breakthrough), and worsening histologic or clinical disease (see Table 6-4). The rate at which resistant mutations are selected is related to prior exposure to antivirals and pre-existing mutations, level of pretreatment HBV DNA, rapidity of viral suppression, and duration of therapy. The genetic barrier to resistance also differs dramatically between agents. Lamivudine monotherapy is associated with the highest risk of resistance, over 70% at 5 years, while telbivudine and adefovir have an intermediate risk, and based on existing studies entecavir and tenofovir have negligible rates of resistance. Cross-resistance occurs within drug classes such that resistance to one agent lowers the efficacy of others within that class. For example, lamivudine resistance mutations also confer resistance to other L-nucleoside analogues (telbivudine, emtricitabine) and partial resistance to entecavir such that interferon or nucleotide analogues become the only effective agents.

Baseline genotypic resistance testing is not recommended when initiating therapy, but once virologic or biochemical breakthrough occurs, direct sequence assays should be performed to confirm the presence of mutations and guide selection of appropriate additional or alternative antiviral therapy. Although minimal data exist to define appropriate monitoring for antiviral resistance, close on-treatment monitoring is sufficient.[25] The recommendation for all cases of antiviral resistance is to either continue the original agent while adding a drug from a different class or switching to a more potent agent within the same class.

TREATMENT ALGORITHMS

HBeAg-Positive Patients

Treatment should be continued after seroconversion for an additional 12 months after HBV DNA levels become undetectable. For those with persistently detectable HBV DNA, treatment should be continued for 6 months after seroconversion then treatment may be stopped in patients with no evidence of cirrhosis, but they should be closely monitored for progression of disease and reversion to HBeAg seropositivity. For patients who fail to seroconvert on therapy, it is recommended to continue treatment long term as the rate of seroconversion increases with time and there is a high risk of recurring viremia (Table 6-6).

HBeAg-Negative Patients

The majority of seronegative patients have lower baseline DNA levels but a higher risk for disease progression so the virologic threshold for starting

Table 6-6

How to Treat Patients With
HBeAg-Positive Chronic Hepatitis B Virus

HBV DNA	ALT	TREATMENT OPTIONS
<20,000	Normal	No treatment Monitor every 6 to 12 months Consider therapy with histologic disease or clinical cirrhosis
>20,000	Normal	Monitor every 6 months Consider liver biopsy; if histologic disease, treat If treated, entecavir, tenofovir, PEG-IFN preferred
>20,000	Elevated	Treat with entecavir, tenofovir, or PEG-IFN

therapy is lower: DNA >2000 IU/mL. The optimal duration of therapy is less clear in HBeAg-negative patients, and HBV DNA suppression and ALT normalization are the only means to assess response to therapy. Patients on treatment should have their labs monitored every 6 months. Long-term antiviral therapy is necessary in most cases given exceedingly high rates of relapse after treatment withdrawal. Hence, it is important to counsel HBeAg-negative patients that treatment initiation is a lifelong commitment (Table 6-7).

MONITORING PATIENTS NOT ON TREATMENT

Patients with CHB who are not candidates for therapy still require close monitoring and follow up. HBeAg-positive patients with elevated viral load but normal ALT levels should have HBV DNA and ALT testing every 3 to 6 months. If ALT rises to between 1 to 2x ULN, recheck every 1 to 3 months, consider liver biopsy if high risk, and consider treatment if biopsy is concerning. If ALT >2x ULN for 3 to 6 months, biopsy is indicated. For inactive HBsAg carriers, monitor ALT every 3 months for the first year, and if persistently normal, monitor ALT every 6 to 12 months. If ALT >1 to

Table 6-7

How to Treat Patients With
HBeAg-Negative Chronic Hepatitis B Virus

HBV DNA	ALT	TREATMENT OPTIONS
<2000	Normal	No treatment; majority are inactive HBsAg carriers Monitor every 6 to 12 months Consider therapy with histologic disease or clinical cirrhosis
>2000	Normal	Monitor every 6 months Consider liver biopsy; if histologic disease, treat If treated, entecavir, tenofovir, PEG-IFN preferred
>2000	Elevated	Long-term treatment with entecavir, tenofovir, or PEG-IFN

2x ULN, measure serum HBV DNA and consider biopsy if level >20,000. Treatment is indicated if the biopsy reveals moderate to severe inflammation or significant fibrosis. For all inactive and active patients not under treatment, consider HCC surveillance for all at-risk patients.

PUBLIC HEALTH MANAGEMENT AND PREVENTIVE CARE

All HBsAg-positive laboratory results should be reported to the state or local health department, in accordance with state requirements. Health care providers should encourage patients with HBV infection to notify household members, sexual contacts, and needle-sharing partners of their status and urge them to seek medical evaluation. Those who test negative should be vaccinated. All hepatitis B patients, regardless of their phase of infection, should be counseled on ways to decrease their risk of progressive liver injury and seek health care services from an experienced provider. Patients should be vaccinated for hepatitis A (2 doses spaced 6 to 18 months apart), and avoid alcohol, and be referred for counseling if appropriate.

Hepatitis B infection is a strong independent risk factor for hepatocellular carcinoma (HCC), an increasingly common cause of mortality worldwide. HCC is most prevalent in developing countries where HBV is endemic, although the incidence in the United States has nearly tripled over the past 20 years.[27] Adults with chronic perinatally-acquired HBV infection develop HCC at a rate of 5% per decade, which is 100-fold higher than the rate among uninfected people. People who remain in the immune-active phase of HBV infection for a prolonged period of time are at the highest risk for both cirrhosis and HCC, and important predictors of susceptibility include prolonged elevation of serum HBV DNA levels, elevated ALT, and the presence of HBeAg. Genotype C, which circulates mainly in Asia and the Pacific Islands, carries a higher risk of liver cancer. Demographic risk factors include older age, male sex, family history, alcohol use, and viral coinfections.[16] While cirrhosis secondary to any number of liver diseases is the strongest risk factor for HCC, patients with hepatitis B can develop liver cancer de novo. Worldwide, between 30% and 50% of hepatitis B-related cases of HCC occur in the absence of cirrhosis.[28]

Patients with longstanding elevated HBV DNA and immune active disease are at the highest risk for HCC over time. HCC surveillance is recommended every 6 to 12 months for all patients with cirrhosis, those with persistent immune activity, and others at a high risk, including all Asian men over age 40, Asian women over age 50, Africans over age 20, and people with a family history of HCC regardless of viral load or ALT levels. The recommended modality of screening is a combination of imaging and serum α-fetoprotein (AFP) level. HCC is a radiographic diagnosis and regardless of AFP level any suspicious lesion should be investigated. Ultrasound is sufficient for screening in most patients, although MRI or CT modalities should be considered for patients with advanced cirrhosis or obesity, which limits the sensitivity of ultrasound. AFP alone is insensitive for screening, but also nonspecific if elevated. Together, imaging and AFP at regular intervals is an important part of preventive care for patients with CHB and can detect the majority of liver tumors at a stage when treatment with a curative intent is still possible.

SUMMARY

Over the past decade, an expanded understanding of CHB has led to updated and evidence-based guidelines for screening, diagnosis, and management, and the introduction of new and effective drugs to combat infection. Society-based guidelines have been adapted into an algorithmic approach to monitoring on and off therapy yet the decision of whom to treat, at what time point, and with which agent requires clinical judgment based on a number of nuanced factors including patient preference. The key components to reducing the burden of hepatitis B infection include early case recognition, education, and enrollment in ongoing care, which occurs at the level of public health and primary care, and referral of patients who would benefit from antiviral therapy to specialty care. While the consequences of CHB, namely cirrhosis and hepatocellular carcinoma, are preventable with close monitoring and therapy, studies show that only a minority of CHB patients who would benefit from therapy actually undergo treatment. Increasing provider awareness of and comfort with managing hepatitis B infection is therefore critical to curbing the morbidity, mortality, and rising health care costs attributable to CHB.

REFERENCES

1. Lavanchy D. Hepatitis B virus epidemiology, disease burden, treatment, and current and emerging prevention and control measures. *J Viral Hepat.* 2004;11(2):97-107.

2. Centers for Disease Control and Prevention. Incidence of acute hepatitis B--United States, 1990-2002. *MMWR Morb Mortal Wkly Rep.* 2004;52(51-52):1252-1254.

3. Cohen C, Evans AA, London WT, Block J, Conti M, Block T. Underestimation of chronic hepatitis B virus infection in the United States of America. *J Viral Hepat.* 2008;15(1):12-13.

4. Wasley A, Kruszon-Moran D, Kuhnert W, et al. The prevalence of hepatitis B virus infection in the United States in the era of vaccination. *J Infect Dis.* 2010;202(2):192-201.

5. Keeffe EB, Dieterich DT, Han SH, et al. A treatment algorithm for the management of chronic hepatitis B virus infection in the United States: an update. *Clin Gastroenterol Hepatol.* 2006;4(8):936-962.

6. Weinbaum CM, Williams I, Mast EE, et al. Recommendations for identification and public health management of people with chronic hepatitis B virus infection. *MMWR Recomm Rep.* 2008;57(RR-8):1-20.

7. Chen JD, Yang HI, Iloeje UH, et al. Carriers of inactive hepatitis B virus are still at risk for hepatocellular carcinoma and liver-related death. *Gastroenterology.* 2010;138(5):1747-1754.

8. Mast EE, Weinbaum CM, Fiore AE, et al. A comprehensive immunization strategy to eliminate transmission of hepatitis B virus infection in the United States: recommendations of the Advisory Committee on Immunization Practices (ACIP) Part II: immunization of adults. *MMWR Recomm Rep.* 2006;55(RR-16):1-33; quiz CE1-4.

9. Goldstein ST, Zhou F, Hadler SC, Bell BP, Mast EE, Margolis HS. A mathematical model to estimate global hepatitis B disease burden and vaccination impact. *Int J Epidemiol.* 2005;34(6):1329-1339.

10. McMahon BJ. Implementing evidenced-based practice guidelines for the management of chronic hepatitis B virus infection. *Am J Med.* 2008;121(12 suppl):S45-52.

11. Lok AS, McMahon BJ. Chronic hepatitis B: update 2009. *Hepatology.* 2009;50(3):661-662.

12. Mast EE, Margolis HS, Fiore AE, et al. A comprehensive immunization strategy to eliminate transmission of hepatitis B virus infection in the United States: recommendations of the Advisory Committee on Immunization Practices (ACIP) part 1: immunization of infants, children, and adolescents. *MMWR Recomm Rep.* 2005;54(RR-16):1-31.

13. Lok AS, McMahon BJ. Chronic hepatitis B. *Hepatology.* 2007;45(2):507-539.

14. Rotman Y, Brown TA, Hoofnagle JH. Evaluation of the patient with hepatitis B. *Hepatology.* 2009;49(5 suppl):S22-27.

15. Chu CJ, Hussain M, Lok AS. Quantitative serum HBV DNA levels during different stages of chronic hepatitis B infection. *Hepatology.* 2002;36(6):1408-1415.

16. Chen CJ, Yang HI, Su J, et al. Risk of hepatocellular carcinoma across a biological gradient of serum hepatitis B virus DNA level. *JAMA.* 2006;295(1):65-73.

17. Chen CJ, Iloeje UH, Yang HI. Long-term outcomes in hepatitis B: the REVEAL-HBV study. *Clin Liver Dis.* 2007;11(4):797-816, viii.

18. Chen CJ, Yang HI. Natural history of chronic hepatitis B REVEALed. *J Gastroenterol Hepatol.* 2011;26(4):628-638.

19. McMahon BJ. The natural history of chronic hepatitis B virus infection. *Hepatology.* 2009;49(5 suppl):S45-55.

20. Hsu YS, Chien RN, Yeh CT, et al. Long-term outcome after spontaneous HBeAg seroconversion in patients with chronic hepatitis B. *Hepatology.* 2002;35(6):1522-1527.

21. Pan CQ, Zhang JX. Natural history and clinical consequences of hepatitis B virus infection. *Int J Med Sci.* 2005;2(1):36-40.

22. Ahn SH, Park YN, Park JY, et al. Long-term clinical and histological outcomes in patients with spontaneous hepatitis B surface antigen seroclearance. *J Hepatol.* 2005;42(2):188-194.

23. Mitchell AE, Colvin HM, Palmer Beasley R. Institute of Medicine recommendations for the prevention and control of hepatitis B and C. *Hepatology.* 2010;51(3):729-733.

24. Khokhar A, Afdhal NH. Therapeutic strategies for chronic hepatitis B virus infection in 2008. *Am J Med.* 2008;121(12 suppl):S33-44.

25. Keeffe EB, Zeuzem S, Koff RS, et al. Report of an international workshop: roadmap for management of patients receiving oral therapy for chronic hepatitis B. *Clin Gastroenterol Hepatol.* 2007;5(8):890-897.

26. Lok AS, Zoulim F, Locarnini S, et al. Antiviral drug-resistant HBV: standardization of nomenclature and assays and recommendations for management. *Hepatology.* 2007;46(1):254-265.

27. El-Serag HB, Rudolph KL. Hepatocellular carcinoma: epidemiology and molecular carcinogenesis. *Gastroenterology.* 2007;132(7):2557-2576.

28. Bruix J, Sherman M, Practice Guidelines Committee, American Association for the Study of Liver Diseases. Management of hepatocellular carcinoma. *Hepatology.* 2005;42(5):1208-1236.

7

Hepatitis C Virus

Elizabeth C. Verna, MD, MS
and Robert S. Brown Jr, MD, MPH

Hepatitis C virus (HCV) is among the most common chronic infections in the world. Approximately 170 million people worldwide and over 3 million people in the United States are currently chronically infected. Unfortunately, the majority of patients with chronic HCV are unaware that they have the disease. The majority (55% to 85%) of people exposed to HCV will suffer from chronic infection, and roughly 10% to 20% of these patients will develop life-threatening sequelae including cirrhosis and hepatocellular carcinoma. Therefore, HCV remains the leading indication for liver transplantation in the United States and Europe and is an important clinical challenge for hepatologists.

DIAGNOSIS AND SCREENING

Who to Test for Hepatitis C Virus

Screening individuals with known risk factors for HCV infection, regardless of whether they have abnormal liver function tests, is currently the most common approach to detect the disease (Table 7-1). HCV is transmitted through exposure to infected blood and blood products, and as injection drug

Brown RS Jr. *Common Liver Diseases and Transplantation:*
An Algorithmic Approach to Work-Up and Management (pp 99-116).
© 2013 Taylor & Francis Group.

Table 7-1

Populations Recommended for
Hepatitis C Virus Testing

- Individuals who have ever injected illicit drugs in the recent or remote past
- Individuals with conditions associated with a high prevalence of HCV
  - HIV infection
  - Hemophilia and received blood product transfusion prior to 1987
  - Ever on hemodialysis
  - Unexplained elevation in aminotransferase levels
- Individuals who received blood or organ transfusion including the following:
  - Notified that they received blood from a donor who later tested positive for HCV infection
  - Transfusion of blood or blood products or solid organ transplantation before July 1992
- Children born to HCV-infected mothers
- Health care and public safety workers after a needle stick injury or mucosal exposure to HCV-positive blood
- Current sexual partners for HCV-infected individuals
- All individuals born between 1945 and 1965

Adapted from Recommendations for prevention and control of hepatitis C virus (HCV) infection and HCV-related chronic disease. Centers for Disease Control and Prevention. *MMWR Recomm Rep.* 1998;47(RR-19):1-39.

use is the predominant mode of transmission in the United States, anyone who has ever injected illicit drugs should be tested. Screening is also recommended for people who received a blood transfusion or organ transplantation before 1992, who have exposure to an infected sexual partner or perinatal exposure, or who work in health care. Lastly, all patients who have ever been on hemodialysis (HD), have human immunodeficiency virus infection (HIV), or have unexplained elevation in aminotransferase levels should be tested. Recently, age-based screening rather than risk factor-based screening has been recommended but the CDC with universal screening of all patients born between 1945 and 1965 to attempt to improve identification of HCV-positive individuals.

How to Test for Hepatitis C Virus

When an individual who requires HCV testing is identified, the most cost-effective approach is to first test for antibodies to HCV (anti-HCV Ab), then, if positive, use HCV ribonucleic acid (RNA) to confirm and document viremia. When testing HCV RNA, most clinicians currently use quantitative RNA measurements as the viral load may be clinically relevant in a patient who would contemplate HCV treatment. Traditionally, however, the qualitative RNA test has been more sensitive than the quantitative test (though this is changing over time as the lower limits of detection in the quantitative are now very low) and could also be used to confirm viremia.

In general, when a patient has a positive anti-HCV Ab and undetectable RNA, this can be interpreted as cleared HCV infection. Other interpretations may be false positivity of the anti-HCV Ab or false negativity of the RNA (ie, intermittent or low-level viremia). In this scenario, the recombinant immunoblot assay (RIBA) may be used to confirm HCV exposure (Figure 7-1). For example, in patients with positive anti-HCV Ab/RIBA but negative RNA, the RNA measurement should be repeated on 2 or more instances, and if still negative, cleared infection may be assumed. In patients with positive anti-HCV AB and negative RIBA/RNA, a false-positive antibody may be assumed and no additional testing is needed.

There are limited circumstances in which HCV infection is strongly suspected and cannot be excluded with a negative anti-HCV Ab. One example of such a scenario would be in the case of advanced HIV and abnormal aminotransferase levels. In the setting of HIV or other immunocompromised states (such as hemodialysis), an HCV RNA should be performed to confirm that the patient does not have chronic HCV with undetectable anti-HCV Ab. HCV RNA testing may also be considered for immunocompetent hosts with abnormal liver function tests that remain unexplained after initial work-up or for acute hepatitis since antibodies may take 4 to 12 weeks to become positive.

WORK-UP

Post-Test Counseling

Patients who are diagnosed with chronic HCV should be counseled regarding the prevention of transmission of the virus to others. Patients should be informed that transmission occurs through contact with infected blood, and

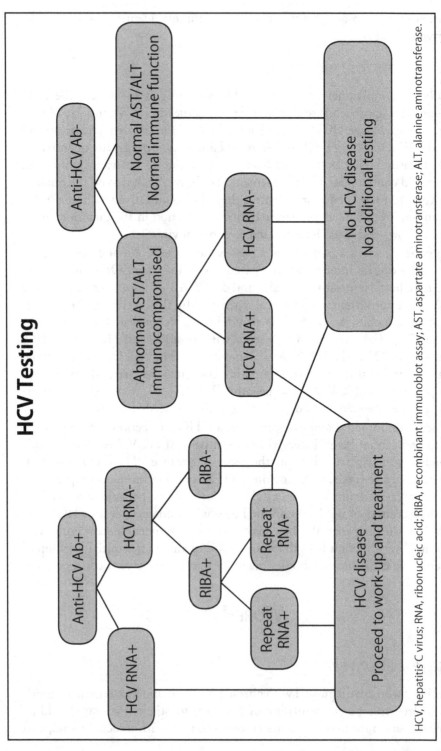

Figure 7-1. HCV testing algorithm. When HCV testing is indicated, the first test performed should be an anti-HCV Ab. In those with positive antibody tests, chronic infection should be confirmed with HCV RNA. In patients with a high suspicion for HCV but a negative HCV antibody, HCV RNA should also be used to determine whether this was a false negative antibody test.

HCV, hepatitis C virus; RNA, ribonucleic acid; RIBA, recombinant immunoblot assay; AST, aspartate aminotransferase; ALT, alanine aminotransferase.

Table 7-2

Counseling for Individuals With Hepatitis C Virus Infection to Prevent Transmission

1. Stop using illicit drugs. For those who continue, avoid sharing or reusing syringes, needles, water, cotton, and other paraphernalia. Clean the injection site with alcohol and dispose of all needles, syringes, and equipment safely.

2. Avoid sharing of toothbrushes, dental equipment, and shaving devices, and cover any bleeding wound to minimize exposure for others.

3. Do not donate blood, body organs*, tissues, or semen.

4. The risk of sexual transmission is low and HCV infection itself is not currently recommended as a reason to change sexual practices. However, having unprotected intercourse with multiple sexual partners may increase the risk of sexual transmission.

* In rare cases, HCV+ organs may be donated to patients awaiting transplantation.
Adapted from Strader DB, Wright T, Thomas DL, Seeff LB. Diagnosis, management, and treatment of hepatitis C. *Hepatology.* 2004;39(4):1147-1171.

advised as to how to avoid spread of the virus (Table 7-2). This is especially important for those with ongoing intravenous drug use.

Hepatitis C Virus Genotype and Quantitative Viral Load

There are currently 6 HCV genotypes (numbered 1 to 6) that can be identified with direct sequence analysis, reverse hybridization to genotype-specific probes, or restriction fragment length polymorphism. The clinical significance of the HCV genotype at this time is mostly limited to type of, duration of, and likelihood of response to HCV treatment (see Treatment Algorithms section on p. 105). It is less clearly linked to disease prognosis. Once the genotype is identified, it is not recommended that repeated testing is necessary unless there is evidence of ongoing transmission exposure. The quantitative HCV RNA viral load may similarly be of clinical use in predicting treatment response.

Assessment of Liver Function and Stage of Fibrosis

Determination of the stage of liver disease in patients with chronic HCV is important for prognosis, treatment planning, and possible referral for transplantation. Only the minority of patients will develop life-threatening complications of chronic HCV but accurate prediction of which patients will progress remains a challenge. Basic serum tests can be used to identify patients with advanced liver disease including the liver function panel, coagulation parameters, and platelet count. Imaging can diagnose advanced disease if the liver appears shrunken and nodular, or if there is evidence of portal hypertension such as ascites or esophageal varices. These tests, however, will only be abnormal in the setting of advanced cirrhosis and may not distinguish compensated cirrhosis from any other stage of disease. Patients with compensated cirrhosis therefore may have advanced fibrosis on histology but completely normal laboratory testing and imaging. More sensitive imaging techniques have been developed including those utilizing ultrasound-based elastography, such as the FibroScan (Echosens, Paris, France), which measures liver stiffness. However, these are not yet widely available for clinical practice in the United States. Similarly, serologic panels are also now used, including FibroSure, FibroSpect, FibroTest, and FibroIndex, which may have some efficacy in assessing fibrosis. These serologic panels are more widely available in the United States than elastography, some including calculations based upon routine tests (such as platelet count, AST, and gamma globulin levels in the case of FibroIndex). However, currently these noninvasive methods are most accurate at the extremes of fibrosis stage (ie, no fibrosis or advanced fibrosis/cirrhosis) and may not be reliable to follow over time, particularly in patients with intermediate stage disease. In the absence of widely accepted noninvasive techniques, liver biopsy remains the gold standard for staging of chronic HCV disease.

The role of liver biopsy in patients with HCV remains debated[1] and while historically thought to be central to the assessment of all HCV patients, as the efficacy of HCV treatment improves, many providers now perform fewer biopsies. Liver histology provides information about both the degree of hepatic inflammation and the stage of fibrosis. It can also be used in some instances to exclude additional liver pathology. Fibrosis is generally scored on a scale from 0 to 4 (the Metavir system) or 0 to 6 (the Ishak system) and may be an important consideration in the decision to initiate HCV therapy and identifying candidates who require HCC screening. However, liver biopsy is an invasive procedure that carries some risks, including significant bleeding (reported to occur in 1 in 2500 to 10,000 intercostal percutaneous biopsies) and death (often quoted to occur in ≤ 1 in 10,000 biopsies).[1] Therefore, biopsies should generally be reserved for patients in whom the results are likely to alter disease management (ie, exclusion of other liver pathology, HCV treatment counseling, or initiation of HCC screening for patients with advanced fibrosis).

TREATMENT ALGORITHMS AND SPECIAL CONSIDERATIONS

HCV treatment with currently available medications, though rapidly changing, remains difficult to tolerate and does not universally lead to viral eradication. Patient selection and education is therefore a crucial part of the treatment process. We know from natural history studies that the majority (55% to 85%) of people exposed to HCV will be chronically infected but that only 5% to 25% of these individuals will go on to life-threatening sequelae of infection, including cirrhosis and hepatocellular carcinoma, over a period of 20 to 25 years. The primary goal of treatment is the prevention of cirrhosis and hepatocellular carcinoma, but identifying those at high risk of these outcomes remains difficult. Excessive alcohol use, HIV coinfection, and substantial nonalcoholic steatohepatitis may accelerate fibrogenesis, and in all patients fibrous expansion of the portal tracts on liver biopsy (Metavir ≥2 or Ishak ≥3) may be a predictor of future progression. Therefore, the risks and benefits of treatment must be weighed for each individual patient, including their likelihood of disease progression without treatment, their ability to tolerate treatment side effects, and the probability of viral eradication.

Treatment Outcomes

The goal of HCV treatment is viral eradication and prevention of the complications of HCV infection. Virologic responses are documented at several time points throughout the treatment period, with the primary outcome being *sustained virologic response* (SVR), defined as an undetectable serum viral load by a sensitive test 6 months after completing therapy. SVR is now widely accepted as being synonymous with HCV cure. Other terminology that is frequently employed includes *end of treatment response* (ETR, virus negative upon completion of therapy) and *early virologic response* (EVR, at least a 2-log drop in viral load at 12 weeks). More recently, due to its prognostic value, the term *rapid virologic response* (RVR, negative viral load by 4 weeks) and eRVR (when the viral load remains negative while on direct acting antiviral agents) has also been employed as it is the best early predictor of eventual SVR. A patient is considered to have *relapsed* if he or she had a consistent negative viral load on therapy but become detectable upon treatment discontinuation. Those patients with a 2-log drop but never become undetectable are called partial responders, while those with less than a 2-log drop at 12 weeks of therapy are referred to as *null-responders*.

Treatment With Pegylated Interferon and Ribavirin

Several treatment regimens are currently FDA-approved for the treatment of chronic HCV, summarized in Figure 7-2 and Figure 7-3 by HCV genotype.

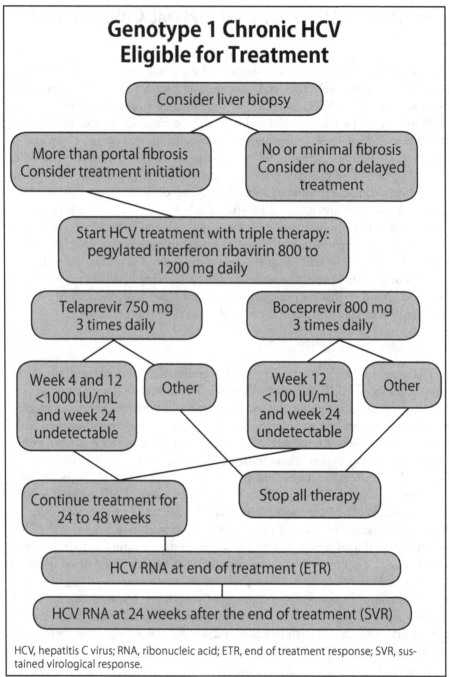

Figure 7-2. HCV treatment algorithm for patients with genotype 1 chronic HCV infection. For patients with genotype 1 HCV and without contraindications to HCV treatment, the current standard of care is to treat with pegylated-interferon, ribavirin, and 1 of the 2 new DAA agents, telaprevir or boceprevir. Treatment protocol and duration vary depending on previous treatment experience and the choice of DAA.

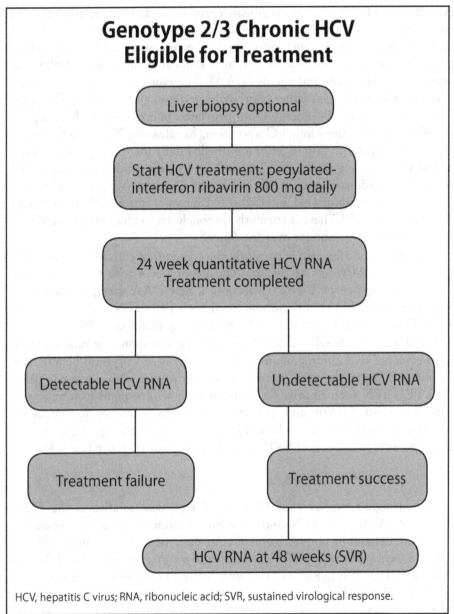

Genotype 2/3 Chronic HCV Eligible for Treatment

Liver biopsy optional

Start HCV treatment: pegylated-interferon ribavirin 800 mg daily

24 week quantitative HCV RNA Treatment completed

Detectable HCV RNA

Undetectable HCV RNA

Treatment failure

Treatment success

HCV RNA at 48 weeks (SVR)

HCV, hepatitis C virus; RNA, ribonucleic acid; SVR, sustained virological response.

Figure 7-3. HCV treatment algorithm for patients with genotype 2 and 3 chronic HCV infection. For patients with genotype 2 or 3 chronic HCV, the current standard of care treatment is pegylated interferon and ribavirin for 24 weeks.

All effective HCV treatment regimens currently include interferon-alfa and ribavirin as the backbone of therapy, but improvements have been achieved in SVR rates in the last decade with the implementation of longer acting pegylated-interferon (PEG-IFN) products that can be used once weekly and now direct acting antiviral agents (DAA). Therefore, the most widely used current regimen includes either pegylated-interferon alfa-2a 180 µg (Pegasys, Hoffman-La Roche, Boulder, CO) or pegylated-interferon alfa-2b 1.5 µg/kg (Peg-Intron, Schering-Plough Corporation, Kenilworth, NJ) subcutaneously weekly with ribavirin 800 to 1400 mg divided daily (depending on genotype and weight) (see Figure 7-2 and Figure 7-3). In large randomized controlled trials, combinations of weekly PEG-IFN and ribavirin have produced higher SVR rates than traditional interferon 3 times per week with ribavirin or PEG-IFN alone.[2-4] There is currently no conclusive evidence that one PEG-IFN formulation is superior over the other.[5]

PEG-IFN and ribavirin is currently the standard of care for patients with genotype 2/3 (24 weeks of therapy) and genotypes 4 to 6 (48 weeks). For patients with genotype 1 HCV infection, 2 new DAA therapies have been approved by the FDA, and are now used with PEG-IFN and ribavirin for 24 to 48 weeks as the new standard treatment regimen (see p. 109).

For those patients who do not have a complete response or relapse, there is no evidence that chronic maintenance therapy is of long-term benefit. For Genotype 2/3 patients with partial response or relapse with a regimen other than PEG-IFN with ribavirin, a small number will respond to retreatment with the most current and potent regimen. In addition, for genotype 1 patients, retreatment with the newly approved triple therapy regimens has a 30% to 90% likelihood of SVR depending on prior response (see below).

Efficacy and Predictors of Response

The strongest predictor of SVR in all treatment studies is the HCV genotype. With PEG-IFN and ribavirin combination therapy, genotype 1 patients, depending on pretreatment viral load, have a 35% to 46% SVR rate with 48 weeks of therapy.[2-4] This is in contrast to genotypes 2 and 3, who achieve SVR in 70% to 82% of cases with either 24 of 48 weeks of therapy.[2-4,6] genotypes 2 and 3 are now therefore treated for 24 weeks in most cases (see Figure 7-3). Genotypes 4, 5, and 6 have less robust treatment response data available, but genotype 4 appears to have SVR rates similar to genotype 1, and these groups are also treated for 48 weeks. Other consistent predictors of SVR include low viral load at the start of treatment (ie, ≤2 x 10^6 IU/mL), younger patient age, lower body weight, and the absence of bridging fibrosis, cirrhosis and/or significant steatohepatitis on liver biopsy. In addition, Blacks with genotype 1 infection have lower SVR rates than Whites[7,8] and there is emerging evidence that Hispanic patients may experience similarly decreased efficacy.[9] Lastly, HIV coinfection also diminishes SVR rates (as described on p. 112 under Special Considerations).

Given the prolonged duration of therapy that is required, a lot of work has been done to identify predictors of SVR while the patient is on treatment. It is now known that of the patients who achieve EVR (at least a 2-log drop in viral load at 12 weeks) with PEG-IFN and ribavirin, 65% to 72% will achieve SVR.[3,10] Conversely, without EVR, only 0% to 3% will achieve SVR. Therefore, prior to the advent of triple therapy with a DAA, this 12-week time point in genotype 1 patients determines whether the patient is likely to respond and should continue to 48 weeks or has almost no chance of SVR and should discontinue therapy (see Figure 7-2). In addition, it was recently shown that over 90% of patients who achieve RVR will go on to SVR regardless of genotype or treatment regimen.

The Role of Interleukin-28 B Testing

Interleukin-28 B (IL28B) is a type III interferon associated with antiviral immunity. Recently, a single nucleotide polymorphism near the IL28B gene was shown in a large genome-wide association study to be highly predictive of the likelihood of SVR with PEG-IFN and ribavirin therapy.[11] Genotypes of this SNP are classified as CC (best treatment response), TT (worst treatment response), or CT (intermediate treatment response), and have now been shown to also predict likelihood of response to triple therapy, spontaneous viral clearance after exposure, and liver transplantation outcomes. In addition, this genotype likely accounts for about half of the difference in SVR rates across racial and ethnic groups.[11,12] IL28B genotyping is now commercially available and can be used in selected cases where additional information about likelihood of SVR will inform treatment decisions.

Directly Acting Antivirals

In an attempt to make treatment more effective, of shorter duration, and better tolerated, several new medications that specifically target components of the HCV viral life cycle have been developed. There are many of these DAA therapies in early clinical testing; however, in 2011, the first 2 protease inhibitors were approved for the treatment of patients with genotype 1 HCV infection: telaprevir and boceprevir. Either of these new drugs used in combination with PEG-IFN and ribavirin is now the standard of care for patients with genotype 1 disease,[13] but cannot be used as monotherapy due to the rapid development of resistance when used alone.

In treatment-naïve genotype 1 individuals, the addition of telaprevir or boceprevir to PEG-IFN and ribavirin increases the SVR rate to 63% to

Table 7-3

Summary of Treatment Recommendations for Patients With Genotype 1 Hepatitis C Virus

	TELAPREVIR	BOCEPREVIR
Simultaneous start of triple therapy	Yes	No
Lead-in of PEG-IFN/ribavirin	No	Yes
Key decision points for HCV-RNA	Week 4, week 12	Week 8, week 24
Response-guided therapy—naïve	Yes (24 weeks)	Yes (28 weeks)
Response-guided therapy—experienced	Yes, prior relapse patients only (24 weeks)	Yes, previous partial responders or relapsers (36 weeks)
Maximum duration of triple therapy	12 weeks	44 weeks
Overall maximum duration of therapy	48 weeks	48 weeks
Stopping rules (HCV-RNA)	Week 4 or 12: >1000 IU/mL Week 24: detectable	Week 12: ≥100 IU/mL Week 24: detectable

79%, compared 38% to 44% with P-IFN and ribavirin alone.[14,15] In addition, response-guided therapy can be used such that the 50% to 60% of patients with rapid viral clearance (ie, HCV RNA negative by week 4 of treatment which is sustained) can be treated for 24 instead of 48 weeks. The approved treatment protocol differs depending on the DAA chosen. For patients treated with telaprevir, all 3 medications are started at once but telaprevir is stopped after week 12, followed by treatment with PEG-IFN and ribavirin alone for the remainder of the treatment course (Table 7-3). Conversely, for patients treated with boceprevir, PEG-IFN and ribavirin are given for a 4-week "lead-in" phase prior to adding boceprevir, and then all 3 drugs are continued for the entire duration of treatment.

In patients who have previously failed treatment with PEG-IFN and ribavirin, SVR rates with triple therapy depends heavily on the category of previous response. Patients with previous relapse have the highest response rates with triple therapy (69% to 88%), compared to those with previous null response (29% to 33%) with partial responders having an intermediate likelihood (50% to 60%).[16,17]

Boceprevir and telaprevir are only approved for use in patients with genotype 1 chronic HCV and have not been studied in many important special populations, including acute HCV, HIV coinfection, decompensated cirrhosis, following liver transplantation, and patients with significant renal disease and/or on hemodialysis. Studies in these populations are ongoing and many new DAAs with a variety of mechanisms of action (including polymerase and NS5A inhibitors), some of which are pan-genotypic, are now in clinical trials. In addition, there are data emerging from early trials of combination DAA, both with interferon and interferon-free regimens, and it is likely that HCV treatment will continue to improve in the next decade.

Side Effects and Contraindications to Treatment

Unfortunately, side effects from all currently available HCV treatment regimens are common, affecting about 75% of patients overall. All interferon formulations available have the risk of serious side effects including neutropenia, thrombocytopenia, hyper- or hypothyroidism, weight loss, hearing and visual loss, tinnitus, rash, irritability, and depression. In addition, most patients experience constitutional symptoms including fevers, fatigue, insomnia, headaches, muscle aches, and "flu-like" symptoms. Ribavirin is also associated with side effects including hemolytic anemia, fatigue, rash, birth defects, and gout. There have been deaths reported in association with HCV treatment due to suicide, myocardial infarction, sepsis, and stroke, and treatment of patients with advanced cirrhosis has been associated with life-threatening decompensation of liver function.

These side effects are generally more common in the early treatment period and are usually controlled with symptomatic therapy, including acetaminophen and nonsteroidal anti-inflammatory agents, antidepressants, and at times hematopoietic growth factors such as erythropoietin and granulocyte-stimulating growth factor. Despite the widespread use of these growth factors by some physicians, randomized controlled trials have failed to prove their usefulness in increased SVR rates and they are not FDA approved for this indication.

Unfortunately, telaprevir and boceprevir add additional toxicities to these regimens. Anemia (an additional drop in hemoglobin of about 1 to 1.5 g/dL) is seen with both of the DAAs, at times leading to transfusion. Telaprevir is also associated with rash, which can occur in >50% of patients. Although the rash is usually mild, it can be severe (involving >50% of the body surface area in 4% of cases) and required discontinuation of the medication in 6% of patients in treatment trials. Other adverse events that were observed more frequently in triple therapy trials (compared to the PEG-IFN and ribavirin arms) were dysgeusia in patients on boceprevir and nausea, anorectal symptoms, and diarrhea in patients on telaprevir. Lastly, there are significant medication interactions between these new protease inhibitors and many commonly used medications. Therefore, careful review of all concomitant medications is needed prior to starting triple therapy.

As a result of these toxicities, therapy is generally thought to be contraindicated in patients with uncontrolled depression, untreated thyroid disease, pregnancy or inability to comply with effective contraception, severe concurrent illness (eg, heart failure, coronary artery disease, pulmonary disease, diabetes, hypertension), history of another solid organ transplantation other than liver (heart, lung, kidney), active autoimmune hepatitis or other autoimmune process thought to be exacerbated by interferon, or age under 3 years.[18] Additional care should be taken in many subgroups of patients including those with significant baseline hematologic abnormalities or chronic kidney disease, and those under 18 years of age.

Special Considerations

All of the large HCV treatment trials were performed with highly selected patients. There are several populations possibly at an increased risk of adverse effects that have been understudied including children, which is outside the scope of this review. Several other patient populations also require special consideration.

Acute Hepatitis C Virus

Rigorous study of patients with acute HCV is extremely difficult due to the generally asymptomatic acute phase of the disease and the lack of specific diagnostic criteria for *acute* HCV. The efficacy of HCV treatment in this setting has been examined in mostly uncontrolled trials and meta-analyses, but in recent cohort studies, the SVR rates are over 70% after treatment for as little as 24 weeks with interferon monotherapy.[19,20] Although these results are impressive, the lack of untreated control groups and the large proportion of patients with symptomatic disease (who are more likely to spontaneously clear acute infection without treatment) cloud the majority of this literature. It therefore remains unknown which patients will clear the virus without therapy, when to start treatment, whether combination therapy is required, and how long the patient should be treated. In general, it is thought that asymptomatic patients are unlikely to clear the infection without treatment and that symptomatic patients may resolve the infection, usually within 12 weeks. Current guidelines state that the high response rate in acute HCV patients "is sufficient justification to seriously consider treatment in most instances after 2 to 4 months of waiting for spontaneous clearance," and that no recommendations can be made about the addition of ribavirin or treatment duration.[18] Additional controlled studies are greatly needed in this population.

Decompensated Cirrhosis

Patients with compensated cirrhosis likely have decreased SVR rates compared to those with minimal fibrosis, but treatment of these patients can often be achieved and is recommended. Patients with decompensated cirrhosis, however, with clinical complications of disease or significant hematologic abnormalities, may be at risk of accelerated hepatic decompensation, infection, and death with treatment. In these patients, the treatment of choice is liver transplantation and because reinfection of the new liver is universal in patients with detectable viral load at the time of transplantation, there is great interest in the transplant community to eradicate HCV prior to the transplant. Given the severity of treatment adverse events in this setting, any patient with decompensated cirrhosis who is interested in HCV treatment should first be evaluated for liver transplantation. Once listed for transplantation, cautious treatment may be initiated often starting at low doses and increasing to the maximal tolerated dose.

Human Immunodeficiency Virus Coinfection

Coinfection with HCV and HIV is an increasingly important clinical problem. Approximately 25% of people with HIV also have chronic HCV, and in the post-antiretroviral therapy (ART) era, liver disease is among the leading causes of morbidity and mortality in individuals with HIV. HIV coinfection poses a number of difficulties in the diagnosis and treatment of HCV. Up to 6% of these patients with chronic HCV do not have anti-HCV Ab, so HCV RNA should be sent in all patients with persistently unexplained liver function test abnormalities. In addition, fibrosis occurs more rapidly in patients with coinfection and HCV increases the risk of ART-related liver toxicity. For these reasons, as well as the emerging evidence that achieving an SVR may reduce mortality in these coinfected patients,[21] HCV treatment in HIV-infected individuals without contraindications is recommended. SVR rates are unfortunately lower than that in the HIV-negative population. With P-IFN and ribavirin combination therapy, genotype 1 patients have a 14% to 29% SVR rate in the largest trials to date while all other genotypes had a combined SVR rate of 62% to 73%.[22-24] These treatment response rates may even overestimate those seen in clinical practice[25]; treatment toxicity is common in these patients and must be monitored closely. Clinical trials evaluating the use of triple therapy with either boceprevir or telaprevir in patients

Table 7-4

When to Refer and Difficult Cases

- Decompensated cirrhosis
- Renal failure and dialysis
- HIV or HBV coinfection
- Hepatocellular carcinoma
- Solid organ transplantation other than liver
- Extrahepatic manifestations of HCV and/or cryoglobulinemia
- Nonresponder to previous therapy

with HCV-HIV coinfection are nearing completion with preliminary data showing improved SVR rates and safety, but these DAAs are not currently approved for use in this population.

Careful examination of the patient's ART regimen is required to minimize adverse effects (eg, ribavirin is not recommended in combination with ddI or d4T). If needed, the patient's ART regimen should be optimized prior to HCV treatment. Patients with coinfection and decompensated cirrhosis should be referred for liver transplantation before treatment. Outcomes of transplantation in patients with HCV and HIV are being studied.

Chronic Kidney Disease

Significant renal impairment is an important consideration in HCV treatment. Ribavirin is renally cleared, is not removed in dialysis, and its accumulation causes a dose-dependent hemolytic anemia. Therefore, though sometimes used, ribavirin is contraindicated in dialysis patients and is not recommended in the setting of glomerular filtration rate <50 mL/min. Interferon monotherapy is the only option in these patients, and the use of ribavirin combination therapy remains investigational in patients with less significant renal impairment. Unfortunately, HCV is associated with kidney diseases including cryoglobulin-assocaited membranoproliferative glomerulonephritis, and is also more common in the dialysis population due to contamination of equipment before screening was possible. Therefore, treatment of cryoglobulin-related disease in patients not yet on dialysis and patients with chronic HCV on dialysis is attempted at times, usually with interferon monotherpy and with modest benefits. This attempt at HCV therapy may be especially important for patients who plan to undergo kidney transplantation, and referral to a specialty center should be considered in this situation (Table 7-4).

REFERENCES

1. Rockey DC, Caldwell SH, Goodman ZD, Nelson RC, Smith AD. Liver biopsy. *Hepatology.* 2009;49(3):1017-1044.

2. Manns MP, McHutchison JG, Gordon SC, et al. Peginterferon alfa-2b plus ribavirin compared with interferon alfa-2b plus ribavirin for initial treatment of chronic hepatitis C: a randomised trial. *Lancet.* 2001;358(9286):958-965.

3. Fried MW, Shiffman ML, Reddy KR, et al. Peginterferon alfa-2a plus ribavirin for chronic hepatitis C virus infection. *N Engl J Med.* 2002;347(13):975-982.

4. Hadziyannis SJ, Sette H Jr, Morgan TR, et al. Peginterferon-alpha2a and ribavirin combination therapy in chronic hepatitis C: a randomized study of treatment duration and ribavirin dose. *Ann Intern Med.* 2004;140(5):346-355.

5. McHutchison JG, Lawitz EJ, Shiffman ML, et al. Peginterferon alfa-2b or alfa-2a with ribavirin for treatment of hepatitis C infection. *N Engl J Med.* 2009;361(6):580-593.

6. Shiffman ML, Suter F, Bacon BR, et al. Peginterferon alfa-2a and ribavirin for 16 or 24 weeks in HCV genotype 2 or 3. *N Engl J Med.* 2007;357(2):124-134.

7. Conjeevaram HS, Fried MW, Jeffers LJ, et al. Peginterferon and ribavirin treatment in African American and Caucasian American patients with hepatitis C genotype 1. *Gastroenterology.* 2006;131(2):470-477.

8. McHutchison JG, Poynard T, Pianko S, et al. The impact of interferon plus ribavirin on response to therapy in black patients with chronic hepatitis C. The International Hepatitis Interventional Therapy Group. *Gastroenterology.* 2000;119(5):1317-1323.

9. Rodriguez-Torres M, Jeffers LJ, Sheikh MY, et al. Peginterferon alfa-2a and ribavirin in Latino and non-Latino whites with hepatitis C. *N Engl J Med.* 2009;360(3):257-267.

10. Davis GL, Wong JB, McHutchison JG, Manns MP, Harvey J, Albrecht J. Early virologic response to treatment with peginterferon alfa-2b plus ribavirin in patients with chronic hepatitis C. *Hepatology.* 2003;38(3):645-652.

11. Ge D, Fellay J, Thompson AJ, et al. Genetic variation in IL28B predicts hepatitis C treatment-induced viral clearance. *Nature.* 2009;461(7262):399-401.

12. Thomas DL, Thio CL, Martin MP, et al. Genetic variation in IL28B and spontaneous clearance of hepatitis C virus. *Nature.* 2009;461(7265):798-801.

13. Ghany MG, Nelson DR, Strader DB, Thomas DL, Seeff LB. An update on treatment of genotype 1 chronic hepatitis C virus infection: 2011 practice guideline by the American Association for the Study of Liver Diseases. *Hepatology.* 2011;54(4):1433-1444.

14. McHutchison JG, Everson GT, Gordon SC, et al. Telaprevir with peginterferon and ribavirin for chronic HCV genotype 1 infection. *N Engl J Med.* 2009;360(18):1827-1838.

15. Hezode C, Forestier N, Dusheiko G, et al. Telaprevir and peginterferon with or without ribavirin for chronic HCV infection. *N Engl J Med.* 2009;360(18):1839-1850.

16. Bacon BR, Gordon SC, Lawitz E, et al. Boceprevir for previously treated chronic HCV genotype 1 infection. *N Engl J Med.* 2011;364(13):1207-1217.

17. Zeuzem S, Andreone P, Pol S, et al. Telaprevir for retreatment of HCV infection. *N Engl J Med.* 2011;364(25):2417-2428.

18. Strader DB, Wright T, Thomas DL, Seeff LB. Diagnosis, management, and treatment of hepatitis C. *Hepatology.* 2004;39(4):1147-1171.

19. Jaeckel E, Cornberg M, Wedemeyer H, et al. Treatment of acute hepatitis C with interferon alfa-2b. *N Engl J Med.* 2001;345(20):1452-1457.

20. Wiegand J, Buggisch P, Boecher W, et al. Early monotherapy with pegylated interferon alpha-2b for acute hepatitis C infection: the HEP-NET acute-HCV-II study. *Hepatology.* 2006;43(2):250-256.

21. Berenguer J, Alvarez-Pellicer J, Martin PM, et al. Sustained virological response to interferon plus ribavirin reduces liver-related complications and mortality in patients coinfected with human immunodeficiency virus and hepatitis C virus. *Hepatology.* 2009;50(2):407-413.

22. Chung RT, Andersen J, Volberding P, et al. Peginterferon Alfa-2a plus ribavirin versus interferon alfa-2a plus ribavirin for chronic hepatitis C in HIV-coinfected persons. *N Engl J Med.* 2004;351(5):451-459.

23. Torriani FJ, Rodriguez-Torres M, Rockstroh JK, et al. Peginterferon Alfa-2a plus ribavirin for chronic hepatitis C virus infection in HIV-infected patients. *N Engl J Med.* 2004;351(5):438-450.

24. Carrat F, Bani-Sadr F, Pol S, et al. Pegylated interferon alfa-2b vs standard interferon alfa-2b, plus ribavirin, for chronic hepatitis C in HIV-infected patients: a randomized controlled trial. *JAMA.* 2004;292(23):2839-2848.

25. Mehta SH, Lucas GM, Mirel LB, et al. Limited effectiveness of antiviral treatment for hepatitis C in an urban HIV clinic. *AIDS.* 2006;20(18):2361-2369.

26. Recommendations for prevention and control of hepatitis C virus (HCV) infection and HCV-related chronic disease. Centers for Disease Control and Prevention. *MMWR Recomm Rep.* 1998;47(RR-19):1-39.

8

Alcoholic and Nonalcoholic Fatty Liver Disease

Scott A. Fink, MD, MPH, FACP

Alcoholic liver disease and nonalcoholic liver disease both represent spectrums of liver disease united by similar patterns of progression and pathology but are divided by different inciting factors. Alcohol can induce hepatic steatosis in a subset of the population. In nonalcoholic fatty liver disease (NAFLD), insulin resistance contributes to the development of hepatic steatosis. Both processes can in turn lead to inflammatory changes among hepatocytes followed by progression of fibrosis until the liver becomes cirrhotic.

The spectrum of disease in both alcoholic and nonalcoholic liver disease forges a common pathway regardless of whether alcohol or obesity/insulin resistance is the initial insult. In both cases, an initial state of hepatic steatosis is followed by an inflammatory state (nonalcoholic steatohepatitis or alcoholic hepatitis). Continuing inflammation induces hepatic fibrosis. Fibrosis eventually overwhelms the liver's ability to repair itself and cirrhosis ensues.

This chapter will focus on the screening, diagnosis, and treatment of alcoholic and nonalcoholic fatty liver disease. Table 8-1 and Table 8-2 summarize the differences and management of alcoholic and nonalcoholic fatty liver disease.

Brown RS Jr. *Common Liver Diseases and Transplantation:*
An Algorithmic Approach to Work-Up and Management (pp 117-129).
© 2013 Taylor & Francis Group.

Table 8-1

Key Features of Alcoholic Fatty Liver Disease

- The risk for developing cirrhosis as a consequence of alcohol use begins with the consumption of greater than 30 g of alcohol per day
- The CAGE questionnaire can help identify patients with alcohol dependency
- The relationship between the amount of alcohol ingested and the risk of developing alcoholic liver disease is not linear
- The generation of free radicals during oxidative reduction in the metabolism of alcohol can induce inflammation and damage hepatocytes
- Alcoholic hepatitis is a clinical syndrome of acute jaundice and liver dysfunction
- The pathologic hallmarks of alcoholic liver disease are ballooned hepatocytes, Mallory bodies, and macrosteatosis
- Characteristically, patients with alcoholic hepatitis have an AST:ALT ratio greater than 2
- A Maddrey discriminant function score greater than 32 indicates a poor prognosis and the need for therapy with corticosteroids
- Pentoxyfylline also has benefits in the treatment of alcoholic hepatitis
- Patients with a MELD score greater than 10, a Child-Pugh score greater than 7, or any portal hypertensive complication should be referred to a transplant hepatologist for evaluation

ALCOHOLIC LIVER DISEASE

Screening

Alcohol use is responsible for 2.3 million years of life lost in the United States and is the third leading preventable cause of death.[1] Two-thirds of adult Americans drink alcohol on a regular basis. The risk for developing cirrhosis begins at the threshold value of consumption of more than 30 g of alcohol per day and is highest among consumers of 120 g of alcohol per day.[2] Alcohol consumption contributes at least in part to greater than 40% of all deaths from liver disease.

Alcohol dependence is defined as excessive drinking and the development of physical tolerance and withdrawal symptoms. Alcohol abuse, or "problem

Table 8-2

Key Features of Nonalcoholic Fatty Liver Disease

- NASH describes cases of steatohepatitis in the context of steatosis while NAFLD describes all patients with steatosis regardless of whether they have steatohepatitis or not
- The pathogenesis of NASH involves "2 hits": steatosis and oxidative stress
- Hepatic steatosis is a direct consequence of the metabolic syndrome
- NAFLD is defined by the presence of steatosis in greater than 30% of hepatic lobules
- NASH is pathologically indistinguishable from alcoholic hepatitis
- NASH can lead to cirrhosis
- NAFLD increases the risk for hepatocellular carcinoma
- Numerous agents have been tried in the treatment of NASH with hypoglycemic agents such as thiazolinediones and metformin showing the most promise and vitamin E therapy having been shown to be associated with histologic improvement
- Diet, weight loss, and glycemic control in patients with diabetes remain the mainstay of therapy

drinking," occurs when drinkers engage in harmful uses of alcohol and consequently leads to negative health and social consequences. Using these criteria, 4% to 8% of the United States population meets the criteria for alcohol use or dependence.

The first step, then, in diagnosing alcoholic liver disease is to better understand how much an individual drinks. One tool used to ascertain whether patients are dependent on or abuse alcohol is the CAGE questionnaire.[3] This questionnaire consists of 4 simple questions. Answering "yes" to 2 or more questions indicates clinically significant drinking while higher scores are indicative of alcohol-related problems. The questions include the following:

1. Have you ever felt you should cut down on your drinking?

2. Have people annoyed you by criticizing your drinking?

3. Have you ever felt bad or guilty about your drinking?

4. Have you ever had a drink the first thing in the morning to steady your nerves or to get rid of a hangover (eye-opener)?

The relationship between the amount of alcohol ingested and the risk of developing alcoholic liver disease is not linear. The risk of cirrhosis increases with ingestion of greater than 60 to 80 g of alcohol per day in men and greater than 20 g/day in women for at least 10 years. As a point of reference, the standard drink in the United States has 12 g of alcohol. Less than half of patients who drink alcohol at these levels, however, go on to develop cirrhosis. There does seem to be a synergistic relationship between viral hepatitis and alcohol in terms of liver disease progression.

Ethanol is converted to acetaldehyde in the cytosol of the hepatocyte by means of an oxidation-reduction reaction. The acetaldehyde is then converted to acetate which is released into the circulation; it is acetaldehyde that is responsible for some of the untoward effects of ethanol intoxication such as dizziness and nausea. Important in this process is that the oxidation-reduction reactions lead to the production of harmful reactive oxygen species that can damage the hepatocyte and induce inflammation.

Meanwhile, in the intestine ethanol causes the translocation of lipopolysaccharide (endotoxin) from the small intestine into the portal vein where it is transported to the liver. There, lipopolysaccharide activates Kupffer cells leading to the generation of cytokines and additional reactive oxygen species that contribute to the liver damage.[4]

The net result of these processes is direct hepatocyte damage and a stimulation of inflammation through cytokine and lipopolysaccharide-induced activation of Kupffer cells. Additionally, hepatic steatosis from alcohol use further complicates matters by acting as a substrate for inflammation. Continuing inflammation and Kupffer cell activation leads to fibrosis and, in time, cirrhosis.

Diagnosis

Alcoholic liver disease presents usually as either alcoholic hepatitis or cirrhosis. We will focus primarily on the diagnosis and treatment of alcoholic hepatitis.

Alcoholic hepatitis is a clinical syndrome of acute jaundice and liver dysfunction that usually occurs after long-term alcohol use. It is an inflammatory process; fibrosis is usually present but patients may not be cirrhotic. Portal hypertension may occur as a result of macrovascular occlusion secondary to hepatic swelling.

The presentation of alcoholic hepatitis is characterized by the rapid onset of jaundice, fever, ascites, proximal muscle loss (usually indicative of longstanding disease), encephalopathy, and the presence of an enlarged and tender liver.

On physical examination, patients may have signs of chronic alcohol use including parotid gland enlargement, Dupuytren's contractures, and gynecomastia. In cases of severe liver disease, the clinician may see visible veins across the abdominal wall, edema and anasarca, spider telangiectasiae, and ascites. Characteristic of alcoholic hepatitis, the clinician may sometimes hear a hepatic bruit upon auscultation of the liver.

Microscopically, the liver shows ballooned (swollen) hepatocytes, Mallory bodies (amorphous eosinophilic inclusion bodies) surrounded by neutrophils, and the presence in hepatocytes of large fat globules (macrosteatosis).[2]

On laboratory examination, the hallmark of alcoholic hepatitis is a characteristic elevation of serum aminotransferases. Classically, one sees an AST:ALT ratio greater than 2. This is a consequence of alcohol-induced depletion of hepatic pyridoxal 5'-phosphate, which leads to reduced levels of ALT in alcoholic patients. The AST and ALT elevation will rarely exceed 250 IU/mL and never exceed 500 in the absence of other injuries (eg, excess acetaminophen or ischemia).

Maddrey et al developed the discriminant function to determine those patients who present with a poor prognosis and who would benefit from therapy with corticosteroids.[5] The formula is as follows:

Maddrey discriminant function = 4.6 (patient's prothrombin time - control prothrombin time) + total bilirubin (mg/dL)

Patients with a discriminant function of 32 or higher or any degree of encephalopathy have poor prognoses and would benefit from corticosteroid therapy if they do not have the complicating conditions of sepsis or gastrointestinal bleeding.

Oftentimes, the patient who presents acutely jaundiced with elevated aminotransferases creates a diagnostic dilemma for the clinician. Chief among the differential diagnoses of such patients are both alcoholic hepatitis and acute cholecystitis. In some cases, a patient with alcoholic hepatitis is sent for an unneeded cholecystectomy, particularly if gallstones are seen on imaging. Given the presence of significant underlying diagnosis, the rate of morbidity and mortality in this scenario is significant. Fortunately, the true diagnosis can be clarified after carefully examining the patient's history and laboratory testing. Finally, imaging will usually be quite different in both cases.

The patient with alcoholic hepatitis usually presents with a history of alcohol use. The amounts ingested may vary considerably but the absence of a pattern of either recent high alcohol use or a chronic habit of alcohol use makes alcoholic hepatitis less likely.

Patients with acute cholecystitis occurring in the context of cholelithiasis usually present with a history of biliary colic-acute right upper quadrant pain happening in characteristic pattern. Cholecystitis patients often present with fever and chills. The patient with alcoholic hepatitis could have little to no prodrome and may simply present with jaundice and malaise. Importantly, severe, sharp right upper quadrant pain is not a characteristic of alcoholic hepatitis.

The patient's chemistries can also help differentiate between alcoholic hepatitis and acute cholecystitis. An AST that is at least double the ALT is supportive of a diagnosis of alcoholic hepatitis. Moreover, patients with alcoholic hepatitis can present with a jaundice that is far more severe than that seen in acute cholecystitis with dramatic elevations in bilirubin. In the absence of dilated ducts, an approach of waiting with or without antibiotics is warranted in a patient with gallstones, jaundice, and no clear evidence of choledocholithiasis or cholangitis.

Finally, the examination of the patient with alcoholic hepatitis may be different than that of the patient with acute cholecystitis. In severe cases of alcoholic hepatitis, the patients can present with portal hypertension. They may be encephalopathic and have abdominal ascites. Such features are not seen in acute cholecystitis, though confusion can be seen with cholangitis ± sepsis.

Treatment

The first line of therapy of alcoholic liver disease is abstinence from alcohol, which may lead to a complete reversal in disease in some cases. Aminotransferases may normalize in patients with simple steatosis without hepatitis and in patients with hepatitis, their disease may remit entirely with long-term abstinence.

Patients with severe acute alcoholic hepatitis present the greatest therapeutic dilemma as these patients have very high mortality. As mentioned above, corticosteroid use in patients with a Maddrey discriminant function of 32 or greater leads to a significant reduction of mortality—a 20% to 30% risk reduction. It is thought that the steroids modulate the inflammatory process leading to a reduction in circulating levels of proinflammatory cytokines.

Another strategy focuses directly on mitigating the effects of dysregulated cytokines. Pentoxyfylline, which inhibits production of TNF-alpha and other cytokines, results in a 40% reduction in in-hospital mortality in patients with alcoholic hepatitis when compared with placebo. This benefit appears to be due to decreasing the risk of renal dysfunction; thus, its use may be limited to milder cases with preserved renal function.

Corticosteroids, however, remain the first-line therapy in a patient with a high discriminant function. Other considerations, such as an active infection, may come into play. When corticosteroids are given, they are usually dispensed with prednisone at a dose of 40 mg/day for 1 month followed by discontinuation or taper. Corticosteroids have never been studied in combination with pentoxyfylline but are used in combination at some centers as the additional risk of pentoxyfylline is small.

The discussion of the care of the cirrhotic patient is discussed elsewhere. Not all cirrhotic patients with alcoholic liver disease have had an episode of alcoholic hepatitis. In the case of the patient with alcoholic liver disease, complete abstinence from alcohol use is of prime importance. It is a nearly universal requirement of transplant programs in the United States that patients be abstinent of alcohol for at least 6 months prior to being evaluated or listed for transplant. The requirements vary between individual programs.

When to Refer the Patient With Alcoholic Liver Disease

The patient with cirrhosis and end-stage liver disease who is abstinent of alcohol and a candidate for liver transplantation should be referred to a transplant hepatologist as soon as possible to begin liver transplant evaluation. Generally, a Model for End-Stage Liver Disease (MELD) score above 10, a Child-Pugh score over 7, any portal hypertensive complication, and a lesion compatible with HCC are all indications for transplantation. At this stage in the disease, there is no alternative therapy outside of liver transplant and expeditious referral of abstinent patients is of utmost importance.

Patients with acute alcoholic hepatitis should also be referred to a hepatologist or general gastroenterologist to best assess whether the patient should be treated with corticosteroids. Transplantation is generally contraindicated with acute alcoholic hepatitis, though this is controversial particularly in Europe.

NONALCOHOLIC FATTY LIVER DISEASE

Overview

Roughly two-thirds of American adults are overweight as defined by a body mass index (BMI) ≥25.[6] Of adults over age 20, 64.5 million (61.9%) and 65.1 million (67.2%) are overweight. Nearly one-third of all adults are obese as defined by having a BMI ≥30. Thus, a minority of American adults has a healthy body weight as defined by a BMI ≥18.5 but <25.

From 1960 to 2000, the prevalence of obesity more than doubled from 13.3% to 30.9% of the population.[7] The percentage of individuals defined as overweight jumped from 31.5% to 33.6%.[8] Perhaps most striking is the fact that in 1991 only 4 states had obesity rates of 15% or higher while in 2000 every state except Colorado had obesity rates of 15% or more. The total cost of the epidemic of overweight and obesity to the United States economy has been estimated to be $117 billion.[9]

While associations between non-insulin-dependent diabetes mellitus (NIDDM), hepatic steatosis, and obesity have been long noted, the distillation of the role that obesity plays in liver disease has only been appreciated over the past 30 years. The first cases of fatty liver disease resembling alcoholic hepatitis in the United States were described by Adler and Schaffner and appeared in the literature in 1979.[10,11] Ludwig et al coined the phrase *nonalcoholic steatohepatitis* (NASH) to describe the "hitherto unnamed" disease.[12] NASH describes histologically defined cases of steatohepatitis with characteristic elements of steatosis and injury while NAFLD includes the full range of liver disorders associated with hepatic steatosis.

Estimates of the prevalence of NAFLD and NASH range from 3% to 30%.[10] One study noted NASH as the reason for evaluation for orthotopic liver transplantation (OLT) in 2.6% of their patients.[13]

The pathogenesis of NASH involves "2 hits" with the "hits" being steatosis and oxidative stress.[14] Oxidative stress generates harmful free radicals that react with steatotic hepatocytes leading to hepatocellular injury. Inflammation, hepatic stellate cell activation, and fibrosis ensue.

Steatosis is a direct effect of the insulin resistance or metabolic syndrome. Also known as syndrome X, insulin resistance is associated with impaired glucose metabolism and fatty acid utilization, dyslipidemia, and a resulting inflammatory state that can lead to a steatosis-inducing cascade of cytokines, hormones, and growth factors ultimately leading to deposition of lipid in the liver.[15] The World Health Organization has set criteria of hyperinsulinemia, abdominal obesity, dyslipidemia, and hypertension as a definition of the metabolic syndrome.[16]

NAFLD and obesity are clearly of immense importance to the hepatologist. Utilizing data from the current trends in obesity, estimates have been made of the future numbers of liver transplants that will need to be performed as a consequence of NAFLD. It has been estimated that if 0.002% of the population with NASH will need OLT, then 500 OLTs will need to be performed in 2025 for the more than 25 million projected patients with NASH.[17] In 2002, it was estimated that 160 OLTs were performed for NASH. In 20 years, there will be a 3-fold increase in the number of OLTs performed for NASH.

The term *nonalcoholic fatty liver disease* encompasses steatosis of the liver that is not due to alcohol. A subset of patients with NAFLD will go on to develop significant inflammation—NASH. If NASH continues unabated, fibrosis will occur, which can culminate in cirrhosis.

Diagnosis

NAFLD is defined by the presence of significant steatosis in the liver with greater than 30% of the hepatic lobules being involved. NASH is a hepatitis that is characterized by significant steatosis and is indistinguishable on biopsy from alcoholic steatohepatitis but occurs in patients who lack a significant alcohol history. This is usually defined as consuming less than 20 g of ethanol per week. The absence of another form of hepatitis such as viral hepatitis is also important in making the diagnosis.

The risk factors for NAFLD include those of the metabolic syndrome. Central obesity, type 2 diabetes mellitus, and dyslipidemia are all associated with NAFLD. It is thought that NAFLD is the hepatic manifestation of the metabolic syndrome as coronary artery disease, cerebrovascular disease, and hypertension are the vascular manifestations of the metabolic syndrome.

It is thought that NAFLD is the most common liver disease in western industrialized nations and thought to affect some 20% to 40% of the general population. It is most commonly found in men. The majority of cases are diagnosed between the ages of 40 and 60. Hispanics have the highest rates of the disease followed by Whites and Blacks.

Pathologically, NASH is indistinguishable from alcoholic steatohepatitis and is characterized by macrovesicular steatosis, hepatocyte ballooning, mixed lobular inflammation, the presence of Mallory bodies, and perivenular/sinusoidal fibrosis. It should be emphasized that at the current time, no study other than a liver biopsy can reliably differentiate between simple steatosis and NASH.

On presentation, patients with simple steatosis can be asymptomatic and have normal liver chemistries. Others may have elevated aminotransferases. Patients with NASH will usually have elevated aminotransferases. Patients with cirrhosis may present with all the hallmarks of cirrhotic liver disease. In 90% of patients with NASH, aminotransferases are elevated. Classically, the AST:ALT ratio is less than 1 in NASH and greater than 1 (usually greater than 2) in ASH. The AST:ALT ratio can be over 1 in patients with NASH and cirrhosis but will not exceed 2.

Perhaps some of the best clues as to whether the patient has NAFLD or not is whether the patient carries certain comorbidities, specifically obesity, type 2 diabetes mellitus, glucose intolerance, and dyslipidemia. Obstructive sleep apnea, hypothyroidism, and hypopituitarism may also be associated with NAFLD.

Approximately one-third of patients with NASH and fibrosis will remain stable, one-third will see their fibrosis progress, and one-third will see it regress. Predictors of progression include diabetes mellitus, low initial fibrosis stage, and high BMI. It has been reported that 8% to 26% of NASH patients will progress to cirrhosis. In contrast, up to one-half of patients with ASH will progress to cirrhosis.

A large proportion of patients with "cryptogenic" cirrhosis—those cases of cirrhosis where no inciting diseases can be invoked despite evaluating for the possibility of viral hepatitis, autoimmune disease, alcoholic liver disease, etc—are likely secondary to NAFLD. This belief is primarily based on numerous studies that have shown that the prevalence of obesity is greatly increased among cases of cryptogenic cirrhosis when compared with other forms of cirrhosis.[18] Also, the prevalence of diabetes mellitus is higher in patients with cryptogenic cirrhosis when compared with other forms of cirrhosis.

NAFLD is also associated with hepatocellular carcinoma independent of cirrhosis.[19] Diabetes and obesity have already been established as risk factors for HCC and go hand in hand with NAFLD. In addition, insulin resistance and the ensuing inflammation is associated with the risk of HCC in addition to the development of NAFLD.

For patients with decompensated cirrhosis, liver transplantation is the only cure.

Treatment

Therapy for NAFLD is aimed at improving the risk factors, particularly the metabolic syndrome. This includes weight loss, control of hyperlipidemia, and control of diabetes. Numerous pharmacological therapies have also been tried for NAFLD.

Weight loss has been shown to be beneficial in numerous studies. Weight loss results in reduced free fatty acid supply to the liver, improved extrahepatic insulin sensitivity, and diminished adipose tissue inflammation.[20] Exercise is similarly beneficial. We recommend a goal of a weight loss of 10% of the patient's starting body weight.

A number of pharmacologic therapies have been attempted to treat NAFLD. No trials have involved large enough numbers of patients with adequate endpoints to allow for the recommendation of their routine use. Metformin and pioglitazone, 2 drugs commonly used to treat the insulin resistance of type 2 diabetes mellitus, have been looked at as possible therapies for NASH. One study looking at metformin in a small number of patients (15) found only a transient improvement in aminotransferases and histologic improvements in a very small number of patients.[21]

Pioglitazone, a thiazolinedione class medication for the treatment of type 2 diabetes mellitus, is a PPARγ agonist that improves insulin resistance, glucose, and lipid metabolism. They increase plasma adiponectin levels, stimulate fatty acid oxidation, and inhibit hepatic fatty acid synthesis, making it an attractive drug to study for the treatment of NASH. In a study of 55 patients with impaired glucose tolerance or type 2 diabetes mellitus and biopsy-proven NASH assigned to 6 months of therapy with weight loss and pioglitazone, patients assigned to the pioglitazone arm showed significant metabolic and histological improvements when compared with those patients assigned to placebo.[22]

A larger trial of pioglitazone included 80 subjects in an arm that received pioglitazone. Some benefits with pioglitazone were seen with respect to reduced aminotransferase levels, hepatic steatosis, and lobular inflammation, but the improvements in histology did not reach a level of significance for the primary outcome parameters of histological improvements set by the study.[23] The study also included an arm given vitamin E, which has been associated with reductions in oxidative stress and to be hepatoprotective. In the 84 patients who received vitamin E, histological improvement did meet the criteria for the primary outcome of the study, leading the authors to conclude that vitamin E was superior to placebo for the treatment of NASH.

For now, given the low numbers of patients in the aforementioned and other clinical trials, no pharmacological therapy specifically for the treatment of NASH can be recommended. What can be recommended clearly are weight loss, exercise, and the control of metabolic risk factors including insulin resistance and hyperlipidemia. There is no evidence that patients with NAFLD are at an increased risk for statin-induced hepatotoxicity and these medications can be given in patients with NAFLD.[24] Vitamin E (400 to 800 IU/day) can be safely recommended due to potential benefit and low risk. For patients with documented insulin resistance, we use metformin as it is not associated with the weight gain seen with pioglitazone, though it is also a reasonable choice.

When to Refer

Patients with NAFLD should be referred to hepatologists when they have evidence of developing cirrhosis and require evaluation for liver transplantation. Patients who have NAFLD in association with metabolic disarray, such as uncontrolled diabetes mellitus, hyperlipidemia, or cardiovascular disease, should be referred to a specialized center so that a multidisciplinary approach can be formulated to treat the patient's global metabolic picture.

SUMMARY

Alcoholic and nonalcoholic liver diseases represent similar entities whereby an initial insult (alcohol or insulin resistance) acts as a substrate for continuing inflammation. This inflammation in turn develops into a clinical hepatitis that over time leads to progressive hepatic fibrosis. The end result of this fibrosis is cirrhosis, which is similar in presentation and management to any other cause of cirrhosis. Alcoholic and nonalcoholic fatty liver diseases are indistinguishable pathologically and must be differentiated based on clinical history. The treatment for alcoholic liver disease begins with abstinence from alcohol. For patients with severe alcoholic hepatitis as defined by a high Maddrey discriminant function, corticosteroids may be of benefit. Pentoxyfylline has also been shown to be of benefit in these patients.

For NAFLD, treatment consists of weight loss, exercise, and control of other aspects of the metabolic syndrome. It is too early in their study to recommend the routine use of insulin sensitizers and other agents specifically for the treatment of NASH.

REFERENCES

1. Alcohol-attributable deaths and years of potential life lost – United States 2001. *Morb Mortal Wkly Rep.* 2004(53);866-70.

2. Lucey MR, Mathurin P, Morgan TR. Alcoholic Hepatitis. *N Engl J Med.* 2009;360(26):2758-2767.

3. Ewing JA. Detecting alcoholism: the CAGE questionnaire. *JAMA.* 1984;252:1905-1907.

4. Wheeler, MD. Endotoxin and Kupffer cell activation in alcoholic liver disease. *Alcohol Research and Health.* 2003;27(4):300-306.

5. Maddrey WC, Boitnott JK, Bedine MS, et al. Corticosteroid therapy of alcoholic hepatitis. *Gastroenterology.* 1978;75:193-199.

6. Fiegal KM, Carroll MD, Ogden CL, et al. Prevalence and trends in obesity among US adults, 1999-2000. *JAMA.* 2002;288:1723-1727.

7. Pastor PN, Makuc DM, Reuben C, et al. Chartbook on Trends in the Health of Americans. *Health,* United States, 2002. Hyattsville, MD: National Center from Health Statistics. 2002.

8. Flegal KM, Carroll MD, Kuczmarski RJ, et al. Overweight and obesity in the United States: prevalence and trends, 1960-1994. *Int J of Obes.* 1998;22:39-47.

9. Colditz GA. Economic costs of obesity and inactivity. *Med Sci Sports Exerci.* 1999; S663-7.

10. Farrell GC, Larter CZ. Nonalcoholic fatty liver disease: from steatosis to cirrhosis. *Hepatology.* 2006;43:S99-112.

11. Adler M, Schaffner F. Fatty liver hepatitis and cirrhosis in obese patients. *Am J Med.* 1979; 67:811-816.

12. Ludwig J, Viaggioano TR, McGill DB, Oh BH. Nonalcoholic steatohepatitis: Mayo Clinic experience with an hitherto unnamed disease. *Mayo Clin Proc.* 1980:55:434-8.1010

13. Charlton M, Kasparova P, Weston S, et al. Frequency of nonalcoholic steatohepatitis as a cause of advanced liver disease. *Liver Transpl.* 2001;7:608-614.

14. Day CP, James OFW. Steatohepatitis: a tale of two "hits"?. *Gastroenterology* 1998;114: 842-845.

15. Angulo P. NAFLD, obesity, and bariatric surgery. *Gastroenterology.* 2006;130:1848-1852.

16. Alberti KG, Zimmet PZ. Definition, diagnosis and classification of diabetes mellitus and its complications. Part 1: diagnosis and classification of diabetes mellitus provisional report of a WHO consultation. *Diabet Med.* 1998;15:539.

17. Burke A. Lucey MR. Non-alcoholic fatty liver disease, non-alcoholic steatohepatitis and orthotopic liver transplantation. *Am J Transplant.* 2004;4:686-693.

18. Maheshwari A, Thuluvath PJ. Cryptogenic cirrhosis and NAFLD: are they related? *Am J Gastroenterol.* 2006;101:664-668.

19. Starley BQ, Calcagno CJ, Harrison SA. Nonalcoholic fatty liver disease and hepatocellular carcinoma: a weighty connection. *Hepatology.* 2010;51:1820-1832.

20. Harrison SA, Day CP. Benefits of lifestyle modification in NAFLD. *Gut.* 2007;56:1760-1769.

21. Nair S, Diehl AM, Wiseman M, et al. Metformin in the treatment of non-alcoholic steato-hepatitis: a pilot open label trial. *Aliment Pharmacol Ther.* 2004;20:23-28.

22. Belfort R, Harrison SA, Brown K, et al. A placebo-controlled trial of pioglitazone in sub-jects with nonalcoholic steatohepatitis. *N Engl J Med.* 2006;355:2297-2307.

23. Sanyal AJ, Chalasani N, Kowdley KV, et al. Pioglitazone, vitamin E, or placebo for nonal-coholic steatohepatitis. *N Engl J Med.* 2010;362:1675-1685.

24. Browning JD. Statins and hepatic steatosis: perspectives from the Dallas Heart Study. *Hepatology.* 2006;44:466-471.

9

Autoimmune and Cholestatic Diseases

Patrick Basu, MD, MRCP, AGAF and Niraj James Shah, MD

Despite progress in the diagnosis and management of patients with autoimmune and cholestatic diseases of the liver, these diseases continue to represent areas of significant unmet medical need. While slow to progress, untreated primary biliary cirrhosis (PBC) and primary sclerosing cholangitis (PSC) in a significant proportion of patients will ultimately develop into cirrhosis and associated complications and may necessitate liver transplantation in late stages.[1,2] Autoimmune hepatitis (AIH), though frequently treatable if diagnosed early, can progress to cirrhosis or have acute flares with jaundice and liver failure. The epidemiology, natural history, diagnosis, and treatment of PBC, PSC, and AIH are reviewed in this chapter.

PRIMARY BILIARY CIRRHOSIS

Primary biliary cirrhosis (PBC) is an autoimmune disease of the liver characterized by chronic, progressive, immune-mediated obliteration of intrahepatic bile ducts leading to cirrhosis and end-stage liver disease.[3] Pathologically, the hallmark of PBC is florid bile duct lesions, with damage to biliary epithelial cells ultimately leading to destruction of the small bile ducts. Loss of bile ducts is associated with infiltration of T cells (CD4, CD8), B cells, macrophages, eosinophils, and natural killer cells. There are

Brown RS Jr. *Common Liver Diseases and Transplantation:*
An Algorithmic Approach to Work-Up and Management (pp 131-156).
© 2013 Taylor & Francis Group.

apparent dual genetic and environmental components whereby environmental triggers initiate disease in genetically susceptible individuals. The relative risk of a first-degree relative of a PBC patient is increased 50- to 100-fold that of the general population. Incidence of new cases of PBC in the United States is approximately 2.7 persons per 100,000 person-years.[4] Disease prevalence varies widely by geography, ranging from 19 persons per million in Australia[11] to 335 per million in the United Kingdom[6] to 400 per million in the United States.[4] Prevalence appears to be increasing over time, which may be attributed to a true increase in the number of cases or to improved disease awareness.[6]

This disease predominantly strikes women (9:1) in the 5th decade of life and rarely affects individuals younger than 25 years.[7] Aside from female sex, other risk factors include genetic predisposition and environmental factors such as smoking and exposure to chemical compounds, industrial and/or toxic sites, and xenobiotics.[3] A diagnosis is based on confirmation of any 2 of the following 3 potential criteria: alkaline phosphatase (AP) elevation, presence of anti-mitochondrial antibody (AMA), and histologic evidence of nonsuppurative destructive cholangitis and destruction of interlobular bile ducts.[1] After a diagnosis, approximately two-thirds of patients respond to medical therapy with ursodeoxycholic acid (UDCA); the remaining one-third who fail to respond have few therapeutic options.[3] Liver transplantation is considered highly effective in this patient population, with PBC representing the 6th leading cause of liver transplants.[1] Approximately 20% to 25% of transplant patients will experience disease recurrence over a 10-year interval and subsequently appear to respond to UDCA therapy. Other noteworthy symptoms and/or complications of PBC that require medical attention include fatigue, pruritus, portal hypertension, bone disease, hyperlipidemia, Sicca syndrome, and vitamin deficiencies.

Natural History

Causes of PBC include heritable and environmental components, such that a genetically susceptible individual (eg, first-degree relative has a 50- to 100-fold higher relative risk of PBC than general population) is exposed to an environmental trigger (eg, industrial, coal mining, xenobiotics, infections) that initiates the disease process.[3] The natural history of PBC is chronic, described by a slow but progressive deterioration in liver function (Figure 9-1).[8] A significant proportion of patients are asymptomatic at the time of diagnosis. Disease onset may precede symptom appearance by 10 years. After symptoms appear, it may take another decade before jaundice appears, and patients may live with jaundice another 5 to 6 years before the need for liver transplantation.

The natural history of PBC may be assessed by changes in biochemical markers, histologic markers, and/or symptomatology.[1] Biochemical markers

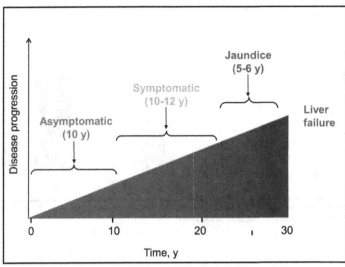

Figure 9-1. Natural history of primary biliary cirrhosis. (Adapted from Lindor KD, Hoofnagle J, Maddrey WC, Mackay IE, Dickson ER. Primary biliary cirrhosis clinical research single-topic conference. *Hepatology.* 1996;23(3):639-644.)

Table 9-1

Liver Pathologic Staging Definitions

STAGE	DESCRIPTION
1	Inflammation is localized to the portal triads
2	Inflammation extends beyond portal triads into surrounding parenchyma Number of normal bile ducts is reduced
3	Fibrous septa link adjacent portal triads
4	Cirrhosis; end-stage liver disease with regenerative nodules

Adapted from Ludwig J, Dickson ER, McDonald GS. Staging of chronic nonsuppurative destructive cholangitis (syndrome of biliary cirrhosis). *Virchows Arch A Pathol Anat Histol.* 1978;379:103-112; and Kaplan MM, Gershwin ME. Primary biliary cirrhosis. *N Engl J Med.* 2005;353(12):1261-1273.

of disease severity (disease stage) include serum AP activity and bilirubin. Elevations in these parameters are frequently associated with disease severity and, in the case of bilirubin, patient prognosis. In addition to monitoring biochemical markers, a biopsy with assessment of liver histology is critical to establish prognosis and, in many cases, to establish definitive diagnosis.

Pathologic stages for liver histology are summarized in Table 9-1.[7] In a large group of patients followed for disease progression, overall the histologic

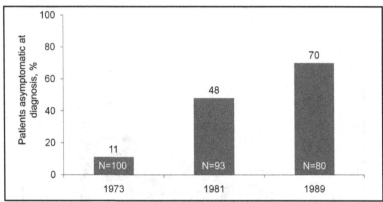

Figure 9-2. Disease awareness and diagnosis have improved over time, with the majority of patients asymptomatic at the time of diagnosis.

Table 9-2

Diagnostic Criteria for Primary Biliary Cirrhosis

Based on the patient meeting 2 out of the following 3 criteria:

- Biochemical evidence of cholestasis with elevation of AP activity
- Presence of AMA: For patients who do not have AMA check for presence of antibodies against major M2 components (eg, pyruvate dehydrogenase complex-E2, 2-oxo-glutaric acid dehydrogenase complex)
- Histopathologic evidence of nonsuppurative cholangitis and destruction of small or medium-sized bile ducts (liver biopsy)

stage progressed by 1 stage every 1.5 years.[1] Clearly, patients diagnosed with stage 4 PBC have end-stage disease and require immediate listing for transplantation.[7]

Signs, Symptoms, and Diagnosis

Patients are often asymptomatic at the time of diagnosis; indeed, the majority of patients are started toward diagnosis following discovery of hypercholesterolemia or abnormal liver function tests during a routine examination.[3] There has been notable improvement in early diagnosis as illustrated in Figure 9-2.[9-12] However, a proportion of patients are symptomatic at diagnosis.[3] Common symptoms at presentation include fatigue in 21% of patients and pruritus in 19%.[13]

Although symptoms such as fatigue and pruritus are common among patients with PBC, they are not diagnostic (Table 9-2).

Additionally, the American Association for the Study of Liver Diseases (AASLD) suggests an algorithm for diagnosing PBC (Figure 9-3).[1]

Prognostic Factors

Although patient prognosis was poor before the identification of effective medical therapy, the prognosis has improved with the advent of earlier diagnosis and initiation of treatment.[12] Parameters that have consistently been shown to be independent predictors of poor prognosis are summarized in Table 9-3. Increased bilirubin has been shown to be prognostic across a number of studies included in the analysis. Other strong prognostic factors (for poor outcome) include advanced age, cirrhosis, ascites, and a decrease in serum albumin. Parameters that have been associated less consistently with a poor prognosis include gastrointestinal bleeding, cholestatic histology picture, hepatomegaly, and changes in bleeding time.

Treatment

The only FDA-approved therapy for PBC (all stages) is UDCA,[1] a hydrophilic, dihydroxy bile acid.[2] Although the precise mechanism of action is unknown, clinical studies of UDCA at a dose of 13 to 15 mg/kg/day have shown improvement in biochemical parameters (eg, AP), histologic parameters, disease progression, and overall survival. Improvements in liver function become evident within a few weeks of UDCA therapy with 90% of the improvement realized in the initial 6 to 9 months. The drug is safe and has no clinically significant side effects; however, the drug has no apparent benefit for fatigue, pruritus, associated bone disease, or autoimmune parameters.

Other considerations for management of patients with PBC include fatigue, pruritus, osteoporosis, portal hypertension, Sicca syndrome, and hyperlipemia (Table 9-4 shows the management of these associated symptoms and complications).[1,12,14]

Although UDCA is a proven effective therapy for PBC, there is ample room for improvement of patient outcomes. Additionally, consideration is warranted to manage disease symptoms and complications (Table 9-5).[1,2]

Several investigational approaches have been tested to date to manage PBC, including B-cell depletion (immunosuppressants), corticosteroids, and stem cells, none of which have yet shown benefit.[1,2]

PRIMARY SCLEROSING CHOLANGITIS

PSC is a chronic disease of the liver characterized by progressive bile duct destruction leading to cirrhosis and a need for liver transplantation.[2,15]

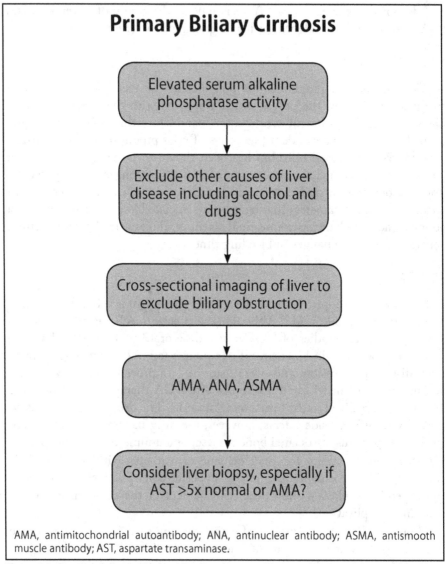

Primary Biliary Cirrhosis

Elevated serum alkaline phosphatase activity

↓

Exclude other causes of liver disease including alcohol and drugs

↓

Cross-sectional imaging of liver to exclude biliary obstruction

↓

AMA, ANA, ASMA

↓

Consider liver biopsy, especially if AST >5x normal or AMA?

AMA, antimitochondrial autoantibody; ANA, antinuclear antibody; ASMA, antismooth muscle antibody; AST, aspartate transaminase.

Figure 9-3. Suggested diagnostic algorithm for patients with primary biliary cirrhosis. (Adapted from Lindor KD, Gershwin ME, Poupon R, et al. Primary biliary cirrhosis. *Hepatology.* 2009;50(1):291-308.)

Fortunately, the disease is relatively uncommon with one new case per 100,000 individuals per year.[15] However, because PSC has a relatively long natural history with a mean survival of 12 to 17 years, disease prevalence is 8 to 14 per 100,000 individuals. The disease is more common among men (3:2). It may present at any age but typically occurs in the 4th decade of life. Initial suspicion of PSC may arise upon finding elevated serum AP on routine examination or in a patient presenting

Table 9-3

Independent Parameters of Poor Prognosis in Patients With Primary Biliary Cirrhosis

PRIMARY PARAMETERS

- Increase in serum bilirubin
- Decrease in serum albumin
- Advanced age
- Ascites, fluid retention
- Cirrhosis

SECONDARY PARAMETERS

- Gastrointestinal bleeding
- Cholestatic picture at histology
- Hepatomegaly
- Increase in PT (INR)
- Mallory bodies
- Esophageal varices

INR, international normalized ratio; PT, prothrombin time.

with fatigue and pruritus[2,15] (jaundice is a late-stage symptom). Magnetic resonance cholangiopancreatography (MRCP) and endoscopic retrograde cholangiopancreatography (ERCP) are the gold standard in diagnosis and should demonstrate bile duct changes with multifocal strictures and segmental dilations. MRCP or ERCP can also determine the specific form of PSC (eg, large versus small duct) and differentiate PSC from other causes of cholestatic liver test abnormalities such as AIH and autoimmune pancreatitis (AIP). Unfortunately, no medical therapy (UDCA, corticosteroids, immunosuppressants) has been shown to slow disease progression or improve survival. The only intervention demonstrated to improve survival is liver transplantation for patients who progress to end-stage liver disease. Patients with PSC have a significantly elevated risk for cholangiocarcinoma (CCA), occurring in up to 10% of patients over time.[16] Additional potential complications include portal hypertension, metabolic bone disease, and inflammatory bowel disease (IBD).[2] Up to 70% to 80% of patients with PSC also have IBD, with ulcerative colitis far more common than Crohn's disease.[17,18] Patients

Table 9-4

Management of Primary Biliary Cirrhosis Symptoms and Complications

SYMPTOM/ COMPLICATION	POTENTIAL INTERVENTIONS
Fatigue	Exclude other causes, including anemia, hypothyroidism, depression, and sleep disorder No recommended therapy, but modafinil may be effective
Pruritus	Bile acid sequestrants (eg, cholestyramine) Rifampin 150 to 300 mg twice daily Oral opiate antagonists (eg, naltrexone 50 mg daily) Sertraline 75 to 100 mg daily Barbiturates 50 mg daily (at bedtime) UV light Albumin dialysis (eg, molecular adsorbent recirculating system or MARS)
Metabolic bone disease	Bone density exam at diagnosis and, thereafter, at 2- to 3-year intervals Calcium 1000 to 1500 mg daily Vitamin D 1000 IU daily Oral or parenteral bisphosphonate therapy for osteoporosis
Portal hypertension and varices	Screening upper endoscopy upon diagnosis of cirrhosis Nonselective beta-blockers for large esophageal varices Endoscopic variceal ligation for varices at high risk for bleeding Distal splenorenal shunt for intractable varices and good liver function Intervention selected on basis of local expertise, resources, and patient preference
Hyperlipidemia	Associated with all cholestatic liver diseases Typically no intervention is required; consider statins in patients with family history of lipid abnormalities

(continued)

Table 9-4 *(continued)*

Management of Primary Biliary Cirrhosis Symptoms and Complications

SYMPTOM/ COMPLICA- TION	POTENTIAL INTERVENTIONS
Sicca syndrome	Artificial tears initially
	Pilocarpine or cevimeline in refractory patients
	Cyclosporine ophthalmic emulsion in patients refractory to treatments above
	For xerostomia and dysphagia use the following: saliva substitutes, pilocarpine or cevimeline, or moisturizers for vaginal dryness

IU, international units; MARS, molecular adsorbent recirculating system; PBC, primary biliary cirrhosis; UV, ultraviolet.

Table 9-5

Principles of Treatment

- A dose of UDCA 13 to 15 mg/kg/day orally is recommended for patients with PBC who have abnormal liver enzyme values regardless of histologic stage
- For patients requiring bile acid sequestrants, UDCA should be given 2 to 4 hours before or after ingestion

diagnosed with PSC without a history or symptoms of IBD should have a full colonoscopy with biopsies, with surveillance colonoscopy performed every 1 to 2 years to exclude colorectal neoplasia.

Disease Features and Natural History

PSC is a cholestatic disease characterized by inflammation and fibrosis of intrahepatic and extrahepatic bile ducts.[2] Progressive loss of bile ducts causes chronic bile stasis and hepatic fibrosis, ultimately leading to cirrhosis, end-stage liver disease, and listing for liver transplantation (Figure 9-4).[15] Although the precise cause is unknown, PSC is thought to be mediated by the immune system, with frequent autoantibodies such as antinuclear antibodies (ANA) and antismooth muscle antibodies (ASMA) and 70% to 80% of patients having IBD.[2,17,18]

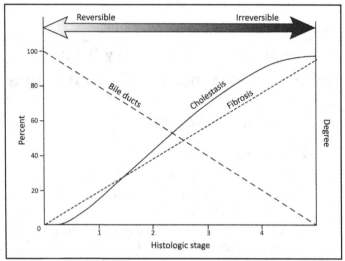

Figure 9-4. Natural history of primary sclerosing cholangitis. The gradual loss of bile ducts causes progressive cholestasis, followed by fibrosis. Early disease stages may be reversible, whereas later stages are irreversible. (Reproduced with permission from LaRusso NF, Shneider BL, Black D, et al. Primary sclerosing cholangitis: summary of a workshop. *Hepatology.* 2006;44(3):746-764.)

Patients diagnosed with PSC may be categorized according to parameters that affect prognosis: asymptomatic versus symptomatic, small versus large duct disease, with IBD versus without, and with features of AIH versus without. In adults, approximately 75% demonstrate both small and large duct involvement; the remaining 15% and 10% have small and large duct involvement only, respectively.[15] Small duct disease progresses slower than large duct disease, and only a small minority of patients (12% to 16%) will progress to develop large duct disease. However, some patients will progress to cirrhosis without ever having developed large duct lesions. As might be expected, patients who are asymptomatic at diagnosis and with small duct disease have a better prognosis (Figure 9-5).[19,20]

From the time of diagnosis, median time to death or liver transplantation is 8 years.[15] Overall, patients survive an average of 12 to 17 years. Because cumulative incidence of CCA is up to 10% and median survival of these patients is <1 year, it is vital to be suspicious of CCA. Although controversial, an algorithm for monitoring PSC patients for CCA is summarized in Figure 9-6.[2] Cholangiocarcinoma may occur during any stage of disease and may be present rarely in patients at the time of diagnosis.

Symptomatology and Diagnosis

PSC has a heterogeneous clinical presentation. Symptoms, if present, can include right upper quadrant abdominal discomfort, fatigue, pruritus, and

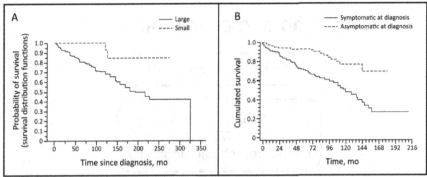

Figure 9-5. Survival among patients with primary sclerosing cholangitis with small versus large duct disease (panel A) and asymptomatic versus symptomatic presentation (panel B). (Reproduced with permission from Björnsson E, Boberg KM, Cullen S, et al. Patients with small duct primary sclerosing cholangitis have a favorable long term prognosis. *Gut.* 2002;51(5):731-735; and Broomé U, Olsson R, Lööf L, et al. Natural history and prognostic factors in 305 Swedish patients with primary sclerosing cholangitis. *Gut.* 1996;38(4):610-615.)

weight loss.[2] Physical findings may include jaundice, hepatomegaly, and splenomegaly.[2,15,20] Other symptoms may include steatorrhea, infections, and vitamin deficiencies. Rarely, patients may present with CCA, end-stage liver disease, or variceal hemorrhage.[2,15] Unfortunately, CCA is a frequent complication that can occur during any stage of disease but is more common in patients with cirrhosis.[2,15]

Biochemical Characteristics

Laboratory testing typically shows elevations in AP and, more variably, increases in aminotransferase levels and immunoglobulin G.[2] Evaluation of elevated AP frequently leads to the diagnosis in asymptomatic cases. Serum bilirubin levels are normal in a majority of patients. Although serum auto-antibodies play no role in diagnosis of PSC, prevalence of various markers (from highest to lowest) are antineutrophil cytoplasmic antibody, ANA, anti-cardiolipin antibody, anti-endothelial cell antibody, and ASMA. Importantly, biochemical and autoantibody markers alone are not diagnostic.

Imaging Studies

ERCP and MRCP represent the gold standard in diagnosing PSC.[2] MRCP is generally preferred in the absence of jaundice as it is noninvasive and avoids radiation exposure but is not definitive in identifying small duct disease. Typically, patients exhibit both intrahepatic and extrahepatic disease and, less commonly, intrahepatic disease only. Cholangiographic findings consistent with PSC include multifocal, short, annular strictures with alternating slightly dilated segments (ie, beading). Longer, confluent strictures may herald superimposable CCA. The AASLD algorithm for diagnosis of PSC is shown in Figure 9-7.

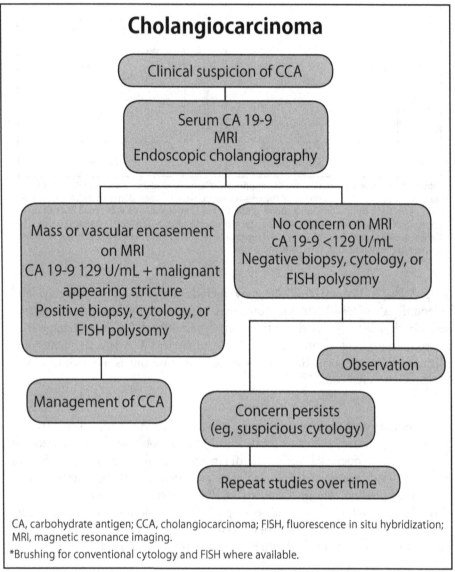

Cholangiocarcinoma

Clinical suspicion of CCA

Serum CA 19-9
MRI
Endoscopic cholangiography

Mass or vascular encasement on MRI
CA 19-9 129 U/mL + malignant appearing stricture
Positive biopsy, cytology, or FISH polysomy

No concern on MRI
cA 19-9 <129 U/mL
Negative biopsy, cytology, or FISH polysomy

Observation

Management of CCA

Concern persists
(eg, suspicious cytology)

Repeat studies over time

CA, carbohydrate antigen; CCA, cholangiocarcinoma; FISH, fluorescence in situ hybridization; MRI, magnetic resonance imaging.
*Brushing for conventional cytology and FISH where available.

Figure 9-6. Diagnostic algorithm for cholangiocarcinoma. (Adapted from Chapman R, Fevery J, Kalloo A, et al. Diagnosis and management of primary sclerosing cholangitis. *Hepatology.* 2010;51(2):660-678.)

Liver Biopsy

Biopsy tissue may reveal periductal concentric ("onion-skin") fibrosis, the hallmark histopathologic finding in PSC.[2] However, the test is not definitive and rarely adds useful diagnostic information. In the early stages, it is not possible to differentiate PSC from other biliary diseases on biopsy. However, liver biopsy is often needed to establish a diagnosis of small duct disease.

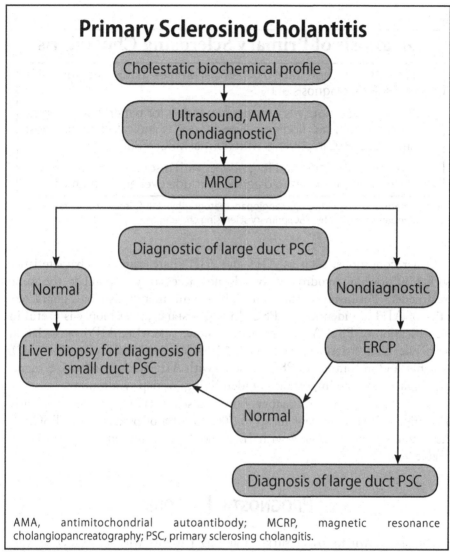

Primary Sclerosing Cholantitis

AMA, antimitochondrial autoantibody; MCRP, magnetic resonance cholangiopancreatography; PSC, primary sclerosing cholangitis.

Figure 9-7. Algorithm for diagnosis of primary sclerosing cholantitis. (Adapted from Chapman R, Fevery J, Kalloo A, et al. Diagnosis and management of primary sclerosing cholangitis. *Hepatology*. 2010;51(2):660-678.)

Differential Diagnosis

It is important to exclude secondary causes of sclerosing cholangitis and to identify PSC overlap syndromes to provide an accurate prognosis and plan for the best treatment. There are numerous secondary causes of sclerosing cholangitis to exclude, including strictures attributed to surgery, trauma, ischemia, tumors, and infections (eg, immunodeficient patients).[15]

Table 9-6

Diagnosis of Primary Sclerosing Cholangitis

- Patients with cholestatic biochemical profiles should undergo MRCP or ERCP for diagnosis of PSC[2]
- Routine liver biopsy is not recommended for patients with typical cholangiographic findings; liver biopsy is indicated to diagnose small duct PSC in patients with normal MRCP/ERCP findings[2]
- Liver biopsy is indicated for patients with disproportionately elevated aminotransferases to diagnose/exclude overlap syndrome[2]

MRCP, magnetic resonance cholangiopancreatography; ERCP, endoscopic retrograde cholangiopancreatography; PSC, primary sclerosing cholangitis.

Other conditions, such as AIH and AIP, share common characteristics with PSC (overlap syndromes) but do not necessarily respond to the same treatments.[2] For instance, the clinical, biochemical, and histologic characteristics of AIH are identical to PSC. In this instance, liver biopsy is useful in identification of PSC-AIH overlap syndrome. Likewise, AIP in association with bile duct stricturing is coined AIP-sclerosing cholangitis (AIP-SC). Notably, and in contrast to PSC, patients with AIP-SC respond to CS therapy, emphasizing the importance of identifying overlap syndromes.

Some form of inflammatory bowel disease (IBD), more frequently ulcerative colitis, is present in up to 70% to 80% of patients with PSC.[17,18] As a consequence, patients with IBD should be screened for liver disease (Table 9-6).[2]

PROGNOSTIC FACTORS

Factors shown to affect survival among patients with PSC include age; serum bilirubin, AST, and albumin levels; history of variceal bleeding; and histologic stage.[15] After a patient progresses to decompensated cirrhosis, the Model for End-Stage Liver Disease (MELD) score is used to plan listing for liver transplantation and overall prognosis.

Management and Treatment

The goals of treatment for PSC include relieving symptoms, improving quality of life, preventing/slowing disease progression, and preventing hepatobiliary and colon cancer.[2] In patients with dominant strictures, defined as a stenosis of ≤1.5 mm in diameter in the common bile duct or of ≤1 mm in the hepatic duct, an endoscopic or percutaneous approach to relieve biliary obstruction may be warranted. Approximately 50% of patients with PSC will exhibit dominant strictures during follow-up. Because CCA is associated with dominant strictures, CCA should be excluded in all cases of dominant strictures. Dominant strictures can induce bile stasis that may result in bacterial infection and secondary cholangitis.

Liver transplantation is a proven successful treatment modality for patients with advanced liver disease. Approximately 5% of all liver transplants are attributed to PSC.[15] In one large cohort of PSC patients who underwent liver transplantation, 5-year survival rates of 85% were reported with recurrence rates of about 20%.[18] The major cause of death in this study was infection. Importantly, patients will still need to have IBD monitored following liver transplantation, including annual surveillance with colonoscopy.[2]

Medical therapy for PSC has represented an area of significant unmet medical need. Indeed, no pharmacologic therapy has been shown to slow disease progression and/or extend survival.[2,15] Recently a placebo-controlled trial showed no benefit from UDCA and actual deleterious effects at high doses. A number of different approaches have also been taken, including corticosteroids, immunosuppressants, and antifibrotic agents. One limitation has been that the disease etiology is poorly understood, making it difficult to develop targeted therapies.[2] For example, although PSC is thought to have an autoimmune component, immunosuppressants have failed to alter the natural history. Additionally, it is often difficult to find patients for clinical trials in rare disease states.[15]

Other Management Considerations

Disease management considerations include minimization/prevention of symptoms (eg, pruritus) and complications, including metabolic bone disease; vitamins A, D, E, and K deficiency; portal hypertension; and IBD.[1,2,15] Recommended interventions are summarized in Table 9-7.[1,2,12,14]

AUTOIMMUNE HEPATITIS

AIH is an intermittent progressive hepatocellular inflammation of unknown etiology. It has a genetic predisposition and females are affected 3.6 times compared to males. It affects all ages and ethnic groups. It may be asymptomatic; however, frequently it could present acutely with jaundice or fulminant hepatitis.

AIH is characterized by the following:

- Elevated AST, ALT, and hypergammaglobulinemia
- Serum autoantibodies (ANA, SMA, or anti-LKM-1 ≥ 1:80)

Table 9-7

Management of Primary Sclerosing Cholangitis Symptoms and Complications

SYMPTOM/ COMPLICA- TION	POTENTIAL INTERVENTIONS
Fatigue	Exclude other causes, including anemia, hypothyroidism, depression, and sleep disorder No recommended therapy, but modafinil may be effective
Pruritus	Bile acid sequestrants (eg, cholestyramine) Rifampicin 150 to 300 mg twice daily Oral opiate antagonists (eg, naltrexone 50 mg daily) Sertraline 75 to 100 mg daily Barbiturates 50 mg daily (at bedtime) UV light MARS
Vitamin deficiency	Calcium 1000 to 1500 mg daily Vitamin D 1000 IU daily
Metabolic bone disease	Bone density exam at diagnosis and, thereafter, at 2- to 3-year intervals Calcium 1000 to 1500 mg daily Vitamin D 1000 IU daily Oral or parenteral bisphosphonate therapy for osteoporosis
Portal hypertension and varices	Screening upper endoscopy upon diagnosis of cirrhosis Nonselective β-blockers for large esophageal varices Endoscopic variceal ligation for varices at high risk for bleeding Distal splenorenal shunt for intractable varices and good liver function Intervention selected on basis of local expertise, resources, and patient preference
IBD	Strongly associated with PSC (up to 70% to 80%)[7,8] Full colonoscopy with multiple biopsies at diagnosis IBD tends to be more quiescent in patients with PSC Surveillance colonoscopy at 1- to 2-year intervals Treat according to IBD guidelines

IBD, inflammatory bowel disease; IU, international units; MARS, molecular adsorbent recirculating system; PSC, primary sclerosing cholangitis; UV, ultraviolet.

- Absence of genetic liver disease, HCV, HBV, HAV and use of alcohol, drugs, and toxins
- Histological features of interface hepatitis with a predominantly periportal hepatitis, no biliary lesions, granulomas, or prominent steatosis
- A prompt response to corticosteroids in most cases

Pathogenesis

The exact mechanism of AIH is unknown; however, triggering agents including infections (bacterial or viral), toxins, or drugs (minocycline, atorvastatin and Accutane [Roche, Boulder, Colorado]) have been implicated. The possibility that foreign antigen mimicry or autoantigen (cytochrome monooxygenase P450 IID6 [CYP2D6]) recognition has also been noted. AIH has a susceptibility to HLA alleles encoding for major histocompatibility complex (MHC) class II antigen (which presents the autoantigens to CD4+ helper T-cells initiating the inflammatory cascade). Certain polymorphisms for TNF-α gene and cytotoxic T lymphocyte antigen 4 gene lead to an increased immune reactivity and disease severity. Miscellaneous pathogenic pathways associated include the vitamin D receptor (VDR) gene, point mutations of the tyrosine phosphatase CD45 gene, polymorphisms of the Fas gene and MHC class I chain-related A gene.

Mechanism of Liver Cell Destruction

Hepatocyte destruction is either through cell-mediated cytotoxicity or antibody-dependent cytotoxicity. In cell-mediated cytotoxicity, the enhanced TH1 response (IL-2, IFN-γ, TNF-α) leads to clonal expansion of cytotoxic T lymphocytes infiltrating and destroying hepatocytes. Certain genetic polymorphism affecting TNF-α production also mediates direct cytotoxic effects. In antibody-dependent cell-mediated cytotoxicity, the enhanced TH2 response (IL-4, 5, 6, 8, 10, 13) leads to B cell stimulation, and hence antibody production and hepatocyte destruction.

Autoimmune Hepatitis Subtypes

AIH has been categorized into 3 subtypes.

Autoimmune Hepatitis Type 1

It is the most common form worldwide characterized by the presence or absence of SMA and/or ANA in serum. Perinuclear antineutrophil cytoplasmic antibodies (pANCAs) (which also occur in PSC and chronic ulcerative colitis [UC]) are found in 90% of patients. The female:male ratio is 3.6:1 and AIH has a bimodal age distribution with peaks at 10 to 20 years and 45 to 70 years. Whites from northern European descent (with HLA-DR3 [DRB1*0301] and –DR4 [DRB1*0401]) are at higher risk. The target autoantigen is unknown, but asialoglycoprotein receptor (ASGPR) found on hepatocyte surface is sometimes found. AIH type 1 is frequently associated with concurrent extrahepatic diseases like autoimmune thyroiditis (12%), Graves' disease (6%), and chronic UC (6%). In <1% RA, pernicious anemia, systemic sclerosis, Coombs positive hemolytic anemia, ITP, symptomatic cryoglobulinemia, leukocytoclastic vasculitis, nephritis, erythema nodosum, SLE, and fibrosing alveolitis are also associated in these individuals. Approximately 40% of the time patients present with an acute onset of symptoms/signs indistinguishable from that of any acute viral or toxic hepatitis. However, sometimes the disease may even appear to be fulminant. Patients usually respond well to glucocorticoids.

Autoimmune Hepatitis Type 2

These individuals are characterized by the presence of anti-LKM1 (liver/kidney microsome type 1) in serum while P-ANCA is absent. Type 2 is seen in younger individuals, usually in children 2 to 14 years old, but can be seen in adults. AIH type 2 most commonly affects Finnish, Sardinians, and Iranian Jews. It is the only AIH with an identified target autoantigen cytochrome monooxygenase P-450 IID6 (CYP2D6) which is found in the cytosol of hepatocytes. AIH type 2 is associated with HLQA-B14, -DR3, and -C4A-QD. It occurs in association with autoimmune polyendocrinopathy disorder (APECED), also known as autoimmune polyglandular syndrome type 1 (APS-1). Features of this disease are ectodermal dystrophy, mucocutaneous candidiasis, and multiple endocrine gland failure (parathyroids, adrenals, ovaries). It is also marked by the presence of numerous organ and non-organ-specific autoantibodies and multiple concurrent autoimmune diseases. As a fulminant presentation of AIH type 2 is possible, all patients who have acute liver failure of unclear etiology should be checked for anti-LKM. Like AIH type 1, AIH type 2 also responds well to glucocorticoids. Patients with APECED and AIH have an aggressive liver disease that does not respond well to standard immunosuppressive regimens.

Autoimmune Hepatitis Type 3

This is characterized by the presence of antibodies to soluble liver antigen and liver/pancreas (anti-SLA, anti-LP). Target autoantigens for AIH type 3 include glutathione S-transferase and transfer ribonucleoprotein (tRNP). It is generally seen between the age group of 30 to 50 years old. The clinical and laboratory features are indistinguishable from AIH type 1. Individuals respond well to glucocorticoids.

Diagnosis

Patients generally present with fatigue, upper abdominal discomfort, arthralgia, Sicca syndrome, anorexia, and pleuritis. Determination of serum aminotransferase and globulin levels (total and fractionated IgG, IgA, and IgM to look for elevated IgG level), ANA, ASMA, or in their absence, anti-LKM1; pANCAs are common in type 1 AIH.

The exclusion of other chronic liver diseases that have similar features is essential. A careful medical history including the use of minocycline, nitro-furantoin, isoniazid, propylthiouracil, methyldopa, or herbal preparations is needed.

Certain new antibodies like actin (anti-actin), asialoglycoprotein receptor (anti-ASGPR), transmembrane glycoprotein on the hepatocyte surface, soluble liver antigen/liver-pancreas (A), and liver cytosol type 1 (anti-LC1) if available also help diagnose patients with AIH.

Finally, liver biopsy is essential to establish diagnosis and assess disease severity to determine need for treatment. The findings of interface hepatitis (hallmark of the syndrome) and portal plasma cell infiltration typifies the disorder, and lobular hepatitis and bridging necrosis (absolute indication for treatment) is characteristic. Aminotransferase and gamma-globulin levels do not predict histological pattern of injury or the presence or absence of cirrhosis. Also certain histologic changes, such as ductopenia or destructive cholangitis, may indicate a variant syndrome of AIH and PSC, AIH and PBC, or autoimmune cholangitis.

Treatment

Indications for treatment are shown in Table 9-8.

Young patients with AIH should receive immunosuppressive treatment to prevent or delay cirrhosis, even if they do not meet treatment criteria.[21]

Therapy in adults is discussed in Table 9-9 and should be combination therapy in most cases.

Monotherapy with prednisone (40 to 60 mg/day starting doses) is appropriate in cases of severe cytopenia or liver failure, or patients undergoing a short treatment trial (<6 months) when the diagnosis is in doubt, pregnant or patients contemplating pregnancy, active malignancy, or patients with thio-purine methyltransferase deficiency.

Combination regimen with prednisone 30 to 40 mg/day and azathioprine 50 mg/day to start is appropriate for most patients who do not present in liver failure or with jaundice as treatment is almost always for at least 6 months. Combination therapy with lower doses of prednisone (20 to 30 mg/day starting doses) may also be used for patients at increased risk for

Table 9-8

Indications for Treatment

ABSOLUTE	RELATIVE	NONE
AST ≥10x normal	Symptoms	No symptoms
AST ≥5x normal and γ-globulin ≥2x normal	AST <5x normal and γ-globulin <2x normal	Inactive cirrhosis
Bridging necrosis	Interface hepatitis	Portal hepatitis

Adapted from Czaja AJ, Freese DK; American Association for the Study of Liver Disease. Diagnosis and treatment of autoimmune hepatitis. *Hepatology.* 2002;36(2):479-497.

Table 9-9

Autoimmune Hepatitis Therapy in Adult Patients

	MONOTHERAPY	COMBINATION THERAPY	
Interval	*Prednisone mg/d*	*Prednisone mg/d*	*Azathioprine mg/d*
Week 1	60	30	50
Week 2	40	20	50
Week 3	30	15	50
Week 4	30	15	50
Daily until endpoint	20	10	50

Adapted from Czaja AJ, Freese DK; American Association for the Study of Liver Disease. Diagnosis and treatment of autoimmune hepatitis. *Hepatology.* 2002;36(2):479-497.

steroid-related complications, including brittle diabetes, postmenopausal women with osteoporosis, and individuals with emotional instability or labile hypertension.

Autoimmune Hepatitis and Liver Transplantation

Liver transplantation is indicated in decompensated patients with hepatic encephalopathy, ascites, and/or variceal hemorrhage during therapy for treatment failure. Patients with ascites and hepatic encephalopathy have poor prognosis and hence should be treated with glucocorticoids during evaluation for liver transplantation, though data supporting recovery in severe cases are limited. Decompensated patients with multilobular necrosis or hyperbilirubinemia that does not improve during a 2-week treatment period have a high short-term mortality rate and require urgent liver transplantation.

After transplantation, the autoantibodies and hypergammaglobulinemia often disappear within 2 years. The 5- and 10-year patient survival rate after transplantation is 96% and 75%, respectively. Recurrent disease after transplantation is common, mainly in patients who have inadequate immunosuppression. In rare cases (3% to 5%), patients can develop AIH de novo after undergoing transplantation for non-autoimmune liver disease. Treatment with increased doses of prednisone or adding azathioprine is usually effective.

Remission is defined as the disappearance of symptoms, normal serum bilirubin, γ-globulin, AST and AST <2x normal, and normal hepatic histology (or minimal inflammation) with no interface hepatitis. Histology findings lag the biochemical remission by ~6 months.

Maintenance therapy is with lowest effective dose of azathioprine, usually 50 to 100 mg/day as a monotherapy. In patients who do not tolerate or respond to azathioprine monotherapy, prednisone ≤10 mg/d can be added or substituted. In patients who do not maintain remission of azathioprine, mycophenolate 360 to 1000 mg BID can be used. It has even been shown to be as safe and effective as first-line therapy in inducing and maintaining remission in treatment-naive patients with AIH, having a significant and rapid steroid sparing effect.[22] Budesonide 3 to 9 mg/day has been used instead of prednisone in difficult cases to avoid steroid side effects. Tacrolimus and cyclosporine have also been used in severe refractory cases.

The duration of therapy should be at least 5 years. Eighty percent of patients relapse when therapy is stopped so many experts use indefinite therapy to avoid the high relapse rate.

Side Events and Management

Patients on prednisone should periodically undergo eye exams for cataracts and glaucoma. They could develop facial rounding, dorsal hump formation, obesity, acne, hirsutism, osteopenia with vertebral compression, diabetes, cataracts, emotional lability, and hypertension. A regular exercise program, calcium, vitamin D supplementation, alendronate 10 mg/day, or etidronate (400 mg/day for 2 weeks and then every 3 months) may help preserve bone density for patients with anticipated steroid use >6 months.

When receiving azathioprine, patients should be monitored for leukopenia and thrombocytopenia. Ten percent of patients have cholestatic hepatotoxicity, veno-occlusive disease, pancreatitis, nausea, emesis, or rash. The use of azathioprine in pregnancy is controversial but it is commonly used in transplant recipients and unlikely to have significant teratogenicity.

Prognosis and Complications

Patients usually respond well with treatment. Fifteen percent of patients may revert to normal histology with complete remission. However, patients are at risk for both complications of cirrhosis and, in cirrhotic patients, hepatocellular carcinoma. Also, complications related to steroids and other medications are to be assessed frequently.

SUMMARY

A summary of PBC, PSC, and AIH is provided in Table 9-10.[1] These autoimmune conditions appear to target different cells within the liver, the small bile ducts, large bile ducts, and hepatocytes for PBC, PSC, and AIH, respectively. In most cases, PBC appears to follow a "dual hit" model, whereby genetic susceptibility alone is insufficient for disease development and an environmental trigger is needed.[1] PBC is primarily a disease affecting women, which has led to speculation about the role of estrogen.[3] In contrast to patients with PSC,[1,2,12] patients with PBC respond well to medical therapy (ie, UDCA).[1,2,12,24] Because patients with PSC have few treatment options, this is a fertile area for clinical investigation. There are a number of investigational approaches for both diseases, including new bile acids, nuclear receptor agonists, biologic agents that block adhesion molecules, and long-term antibiotics. Regarding long-term antibiotics, cholangitis can be attributed to infection by bacteria, fungi, parasites, or viruses.[15] AIH also largely affects women and can present with either an acute fulminant course or a more indolent progression toward cirrhosis. AIH fortunately responds well to immunosuppressive therapy and can stabilize or improve over many years.

With a deeper understanding of the disease pathophysiology, better therapeutic targets and the potential to alter the natural history of disease will emerge. It is hoped that one or more of the newer approaches would delay disease progression and extend transplant-free status, hence improving overall survival for patients diagnosed with these chronic progressive diseases.

REFERENCES

1. Lindor KD, Gershwin ME, Poupon R, Kaplan M, Bergasa NV, Heathcote EJ. Primary biliary cirrhosis. *Hepatology*. 2009;50(1):291-308.

2. Chapman R, Fevery J, Kalloo A, et al. Diagnosis and management of primary sclerosing cholangitis. *Hepatology*. 2010;51(2):660-678.

3. Hohenester S, Oude-Elferink RP, Beuers U. Primary biliary cirrhosis. *Semin Immunopathol*. 2009;31(3):283-307.

Table 9-10

Summary of Features of Primary Biliary Cirrhosis, Primary Sclerosing Cholangitis, and Autoimmune Hepatitis

PARAMETER	PRIMARY BILIARY CIRRHOSIS	PRIMARY SCLEROSING CHOLANGITIS	AUTOIMMUNE HEPATITIS
Causes	Autoimmune; genetic predisposition in conjunction with environmental triggers	Autoimmune; causes unknown; strong genetic component	Unknown mechanisms; associated with infections, toxins, and drugs
Incidence	1.3 per 100,000 per year	1 per 100,000 per year	1 to 2 per 100,000 per year
Prevalence	15 per 100,000	8 to 14 per 100,000	0.1 to 1.2 cases per 100,000 in USA; 11.6 to 16.9 cases per 100,000 in Europe
Risk factors	Female sex Mean age, 54 years	IBD; male sex Mean age, 42 years	Genetic predisposition, female sex, infections, toxins, drug use
Prognostic factors	Serum bilirubin; albumin; age; ascites; cirrhosis	Age; serum bilirubin; AST; albumin; history of variceal bleeding; histologic stage	Age, AIH type 2, cirrhosis, portal hypertension, MELD, complications to steroids
Median survival	8 to 16 years (untreated) Normal life expectancy for early stage disease (treated)	12 to 17 years	10-year survival rate of 89% and 90%, respectively in patients treated with or without cirrhosis

(continued)

4. Kim WR, Lindor KD, Locke GR III, et al. Epidemiology and natural history of primary biliary cirrhosis in a US community. *Gastroenterology.* 2000;119(6):1631-1636.

5. Watson RG, Angus PW, Dewar M, Goss B, Sewell RB, Smallwood RA. Low prevalence of primary biliary cirrhosis in Victoria, Australia. *Gut.* 1995;36(6):927-930.

6. James OF, Bhopal R, Howel D, Gray J, Burt AD, Metcalf JV. Primary biliary cirrhosis once rare, now common in the United Kingdom? *Hepatology.* 1999;30(2):390-394.

Table 9-10 *(continued)*

Summary of Features of Primary Biliary Cirrhosis, Primary Sclerosing Cholangitis, and Autoimmune Hepatitis

PARAMETER	PRIMARY BILIARY CIR- RHOSIS	PRIMARY SCLEROSING CHOLANGITIS	AUTOIMMUNE HEPATITIS
Biochemical markers	↑ AP, AMA, ANA, GGT, pANCA	↑ AP, ANA, ASMA, GGT, etc	↑AST, ALT, ANA, SMA, Hypergamma-globulinemia, anti LKM-1 ≥ 1:80, anti-SLA, anti-LP
Histologic characteristics	Florid bile duct lesions	Periductal concentric fibrosis	Interface hepatitis, predominantly peri-portal hepatitis
Hallmark symptoms	Fatigue; pruritus	Fatigue; pruritus; jaundice (late)	Fatigue, upper abdominal discomfort, arthralgia, or liver failure
Diagnosis	Elevated AP; presence of AMA; histologic evidence of loss of bile ducts (must show 2 of 3 of these characteristics)	Cholangiographic demonstration of bile duct stricturing and dilation; biochemical (↑AP), autoantibodies, and liver biopsy are suggestive	Anti-LKM-1 ≥ 1:80, anti-SLA, anti-LP, liver biopsy- interface hepatitis; ule out other causes; responds to corticosteroids
Treatment	UDCA; liver transplantation	Liver transplantation; no established medical therapy; however, CSs, immunosuppressant therapy, UDCA, cytokine inhibitors, and antifibrotic agents have been tried	Prednisone, azathioprine, mycophenolate (in resistant cases); liver transplantation in 10% of cases (treatment failure cases)

(continued)

Table 9-10 *(continued)*

Summary of Features of Primary Biliary Cirrhosis, Primary Sclerosing Cholangitis, and Autoimmune Hepatitis

PARAMETER	PRIMARY BILIARY CIR- RHOSIS	PRIMARY SCLEROSING CHOLANGITIS	AUTOIMMUNE HEPATITIS
Investi- gational approaches	B-cell depletion (immunosup- pressants); CSs; stem cells	Long-term anti- biotics; cytokine inhibitors; T-cell inhibitors; anti- fibrotic therapy; nuclear receptor ligands	Blocking autoanti- gens, recombinant immune suppres- sors, oral tolerance schedules, and T-cell vaccination Cytotoxic T-lymphocyte antigen (CTLA)-4 blocks activation cascade Autologous and mesenchymal stem cell transplanta- tion, adoptive transfer of T regula- tory cells, cytokine manipulation and gene suppression (small inhibitory ribonucleic acids and short hairpin ribonucleic acids synthesized could match sequences in target genes to trigger silenc- ing mechanisms and modify gene expression)

AMA, antimitochondrial autoantibody; ANA, antinuclear antibody; AP, alkaline phosphatase; AST, aspartate transferase; CS, corticosteroid; GGT, gamma-glutamyl transferase; IBD, inflam- matory bowel disease; pANCA, perinuclear antineutrophil cytoplasmic antibody; PBC, prima- ry biliary cirrhosis; PSC, primary sclerosing cholangitis; ASMA, antismooth muscle antibody; UDCA, ursodeoxycholic acid.

7. Kaplan MM, Gershwin ME. Primary biliary cirrhosis. *N Engl J Med*. 2005;353(12):1261-1273.

8. Lindor KD, Hoofnagle J, Maddrey WC, Mackay IE, Dickson ER. Primary biliary cirrhosis clinical research single-topic conference. *Hepatology*. 1996;23(3):639-644.

9. James O, Macklon AF, Watson AJ. Primary biliary cirrhosis--a revised clinical spectrum. *Lancet*. 1981;1(8233):1278-1281.

10. Nyberg A, Lööf L. Primary biliary cirrhosis: clinical features and outcome, with special reference to asymptomatic disease. *Scand J Gastroenterol*. 1989;24(1):57-64.

11. Sherlock S, Scheuer PJ. The presentation and diagnosis of 100 patients with primary biliary cirrhosis. *N Engl J Med*. 1973;289(13):674-678.

12. Crosignani A, Battezzati PM, Invernizzi P, Selmi C, Prina E, Podda M. Clinical features and management of primary biliary cirrhosis. *World J Gastroenterol*. 2008;14(21):3313-3327.

13. Prince M, Chetwynd A, Newman W, Metcalf JV, James OF. Survival and symptom progression in a geographically based cohort of patients with primary biliary cirrhosis: follow-up for up to 28 years. *Gastroenterology*. 2002;123(4):1044-1051.

14. Heathcote J. Treatment of primary biliary cirrhosis. *J Gastroenterol Hepatol*. 1996;11(7):605-609.

15. LaRusso NF, Shneider BL, Black D, et al. Primary sclerosing cholangitis: summary of a workshop. *Hepatology*. 2006;44(3):746-764.

16. Claessen MM, Vleggaar FP, Tytgat KM, Siersema PD, van Buuren HR. High lifetime risk of cancer in primary sclerosing cholangitis. *J Hepatol*. 2009;50(1):158-164.

17. Bambha K, Kim WR, Talwalkar J, et al. Incidence, clinical spectrum, and outcomes of primary sclerosing cholangitis in a United States community. *Gastroenterology*. 2003;125(5):1364-1369.

18. Graziadei IW, Wiesner RH, Marotta PJ, et al. Long-term results of patients undergoing liver transplantation for primary sclerosing cholangitis. *Hepatology*. 1999;30(5):1121-1127.

19. Björnsson E, Boberg KM, Cullen S, et al. Patients with small duct primary sclerosing cholangitis have a favourable long term prognosis. *Gut*. 2002;51(5):731-735.

20. Broomé U, Olsson R, Lööf L, et al. Natural history and prognostic factors in 305 Swedish patients with primary sclerosing cholangitis. *Gut*. 1996;38(4):610-615.

21. Gleeson D, Heneghan MA. British Society of Gastroenterology (BSG) guidelines for management of autoimmune hepatitis. *Gut*. 2011;60(12):1611-1629.

22. Zachou K, Gatselis N, Papadamou G, Rigopoulou EI, Dalekos GN. Mycophenolate for the treatment of autoimmune hepatitis: prospective assessment of its efficacy and safety for induction and maintenance of remission in a large cohort of treatment-naïve patients. *J Hepatol*. 2011;55(3):636-646.

23. Wang D, Zhang H, Liang J, et al. Effect of allogeneic bone marrow-derived mesenchymal stem cells transplantation in a polyI:C-induced primary biliary cirrhosis mouse model. *Clin Exp Med*. 2010:Epub ahead of print.

24. Poupon RE, Bonnand AM, Chrétien Y, Poupon R. Ten-year survival in ursodeoxycholic acid-treated patients with primary biliary cirrhosis. The UDCA-PBC Study Group. *Hepatology*. 1999;29(6):1668-1671.

10

Inherited Metabolic Liver Diseases

Patrick Basu, MD, MRCP, AGAF and Niraj James Shah, MD

Liver metabolism is regulated by a diverse multitude of enzymes that may in turn be affected by environmental and genetic influences and lead to dysregulation and disease. Several inheritable metabolic diseases impair liver function (eg, glycogen storage diseases may elicit hepatomegaly as a manifestation of an underlying genetic defect), but liver pathology as a primary pathologic consequence of heritable diseases is rare. Three disorders in which one of the main pathophysiologic consequences revolves around liver injury are alpha-1-antitrypsin (A1AT) deficiency, Wilson's disease, and hereditary hemochromatosis (HH). These disorders differ in pathophysiologic defect, clinical presentation, and impact on morbidity; however, liver fibrosis, cirrhosis, and an increased risk for the development of hepatocellular carcinoma (HCC) are common to all.

ALPHA-1-ANTITRYPSIN DEFICIENCY

A1AT deficiency is the result of a genetic mutation within the A1AT gene which encodes for a predominantly liver-produced serine protease inhibitor, eliciting sequestration of abnormal A1AT in the liver and low plasma levels of the A1AT protein.[1,2] The prevalence of this disorder is approximately

Brown RS Jr. *Common Liver Diseases and Transplantation:*
An Algorithmic Approach to Work-Up and Management (pp 157-179).
© 2013 Taylor & Francis Group.

1 in 2857 to 1 in 5097 in the United States, with the highest frequency being observed in individuals of northern and western European descent.[1]

A1AT is the predominant serine protease inhibitor in plasma.[1,3] It inhibits various tissue proteinases (eg, neutrophil elastase) and is an acute-phase protein that downregulates inflammation.[1] Expression of A1AT occurs mainly in hepatocytes, but mononuclear phagocytes and epithelial cells in the intestinal and respiratory tracts also produce the protein. Once secreted, A1AT interacts with neutrophil elastase (not trypsin, as implied by the name) rendering elastase nonfunctional and preventing the breakdown of elastin.

The A1AT gene is located on chromosome 14q31-32.3, and approximately 100 allelic variations of the gene have been reported with the most common being the "normal" M variant.[1] Some of these variations do not significantly affect the processing or functionality of the A1AT protein; however, a single amino acid substitution of glutamate to valine at position 264 (the S variant)[4] and a lysine for glutamic acid substitution at position 342 (the Z variant) result in low plasma A1AT concentrations (ie, <20 µmol/L).[1] Because of an autosomal codominance inheritance pattern, each A1AT allele results in 50% of the circulating plasma A1AT. Thus, the A1AT concentration in patients with 1 of the Z alleles, the most common and severe deficiency variant, is only 60% of that of a normal patient and individuals with 2 Z alleles have only 15% of the normal A1AT concentration. Clinical features of the disorder are variable depending on the specific mutation abnormality and the individual, but lung and liver damage are potential pathological consequences for all variants. Indeed, severe forms of the disease are associated with early onset of emphysema, neonatal hepatitis, chronic hepatitis, cirrhosis, and HCC.

Clinical Pathophysiology

The Z and S variants of A1AT protein are unstable and cannot be excreted from the endoplasmic reticulum in liver cells and form periodic acid-Schiff–positive aggregates within the endoplasmic reticulum.[1,3] Thus, the disease reflects a deficiency of A1AT outside the liver and overabundance in hepatocytes. Individuals with A1AT deficiency lack adequate elastase inhibition leading to increased degradation of elastin structural elements which comprise the connective tissue of the lung.[1] This predisposes individuals to the development of chronic obstructive pulmonary disease (COPD) and emphysema. Liver disease occurs in approximately 10% of patients homozygous for the Z variant and is thought to be primarily the result of A1AT accumulation in hepatocytes. This is because individuals with a "null" variant of A1AT (ie, patients who completely lack A1AT protein) do not display liver pathology, although lung pathology may still be observed.[1,3] In addition, some individuals with Z or S variant A1AT appear to be protected from liver disease

Table 10-1

Clinical Features of Infants With Homozygous ZZ Variant Alpha-1-Antitrypsin Deficiency

- Increased transaminases
- Pruritus, fatigue, malaise
- Neonatal hepatitis syndrome (jaundice, pale stools, vitamin K deficient caogulopathy presenting with excessive bleeding and hepatomegaly)
- Hepatomegaly or hepatosplenomegaly
- Failure to thrive, loss of appetite and feeding difficulties
- Diarrhea
- Symptoms of chronic liver disease/cirrhosis (eg, ascites, pedal edema, liver failure)
- First-degree relative with ZZ variant A1AT

because of a protective autophagic mechanism whereby A1AT protein aggregates are degraded.[1] The precise mechanisms by which A1AT aggregates induce liver injury are unknown.

Children With Homozygous Alpha-1-Antitrypsin Deficiency

Most data regarding the incidence of liver disease in A1AT-deficient children come from ZZ homozygotes in Scandinavia.[1] Most children with the disorder are clinically healthy, but A1AT deficiency accounts for 14% to 46% of children requiring liver transplantation; therefore, infants presenting with clinical features of A1AT deficiency should be evaluated for potential risk factors that contribute to the development of severe liver disease (Tables 10-1 and 10-2).

Adults With Homozygous Alpha-1-Antitrypsin Deficiency

Most individuals with A1AT deficiency are asymptomatic, so the prevalence of A1AT deficiency is probably underestimated.[6] However, symptomatic patients typically present with respiratory problems (eg, COPD, emphysema) during their 30s and 40s. Many of these patients have a history of smoking, so their clinical presentation may not be unique to A1AT deficiency. However, emphysema associated with A1AT deficiency has distinct clinical pathology with predominant involvement of the lung bases and panacinar pathology.[1]

Approximately 10% of individuals with A1AT deficiency develop manifestations of liver disease including jaundice, hepatomegaly, and

Table 10-2

Risk Factors for Severe Liver Disease in Infants

- ZZ variant A1AT male relative with liver disease
- Clinical signs of liver injury: firm hepatomegaly or splenomegaly
- Laboratory signs of neonatal cholestastatic disease with persistently increased bilirubin, prothrombin time, and gamma-glutamyl transferase

occasionally cirrhosis and HCC.[6] Liver manifestations may become apparent at any age, but the greatest risk is in patients >50 years of age who never smoked.[1] The increased risk in nonsmokers is attributable to their reduced development of emphysema and thus longer survival time. The prevalence of A1AT deficiency is 20-fold higher in patients with cirrhosis than that in a normal population. In a study of 31 adult A1AT-deficient patients, 43% developed cirrhosis and 28% developed primary liver carcinoma.

Heterozygous Alpha-1-Antitrypsin Deficiency

Although children who are heterozygous for A1AT deficiency remain asymptomatic, the impact of heterozygosity in adults is uncertain because no population-based studies examining the prevalence of lung and liver disease in heterozygous patients has been performed.[1] There is evidence to suggest that various risk factors interact with the heterozygous nature of the individual and may increase the severity of other liver diseases, including hepatitis infection and alcohol abuse.

Screening and Diagnosis

Screening asymptomatic individuals for A1AT deficiency is not standard practice[1] but knowledge of their condition allows patients to make lifestyle choices, such as not smoking and minimizing exposure to respiratory pollutants that reduce their chances of developing symptomatic disease.[7] In certain instances, screening and diagnostic procedures may be recommended for asymptomatic and symptomatic patients (Table 10-3).

Patients with liver disease attributable to A1AT deficiency display the same signs and symptoms of patients with liver disease associated with other disorders, and other causes of chronic liver disease (eg, viral infection) should be excluded before diagnostic testing.[1] Several diagnostic methodologies are available to diagnose A1AT; however, each has limitations and accurate diagnosis requires use of more than 1 of the techniques.[2] Previously,

Table 10-3

Screening for Alpha-1-Antitrypsin

Screening is recommended in all individuals with a family member with homozygous A1AT. WHO recommends testing in all individuals with COPD or adolescent asthma.

Screening should be offered to the following:

- Carrier screening to all relatives of individuals with homozygous or heterozygous A1AT

- Anyone from a country with high prevalence (greater than 1 in 1500 individuals) of A1AT deficiency, especially Scandinavian, British, Spanish, and Portuguese descent

- Children with more than 2 weeks of jaundice or any signs of liver failure

- Any individual with early emphysema (especially in a nonsmoker or light smoker), unexplained chronic liver disease, or necrotizing panniculitis

- Anyone wishing to conceive who is a carrier or is at high risk of A1AT deficiency; prenatal testing has been available since 1987

- Anyone with a low serum level of A1AT

WHO, World Health Organization; COPD, chronic obstructive pulmonary disease.

measuring the serum concentration of A1AT protein was an accepted diagnostic technique.[1] However, patients who are heterozygous for A1AT deficiency may have normal serum A1AT protein levels, and A1AT levels may increase during periods of systemic inflammation. Thus, A1AT levels should be complemented with phenotype testing using isoelectric focusing or genotyping.

Isoelectric focusing identifies the variant of the A1AT protein present in a patient's serum including abnormal and dysfunctional proteins, but cannot identify null mutations that produce no circulating A1AT protein.[2] Thus, a patient with variant Z null would be diagnosed as type ZZ. In addition, interpretation of isoelectric focusing gels can be difficult and requires trained and experienced personnel.

Genotyping may be useful in patients suspected of having A1AT deficiency; however, current procedures specifically test for the presence of the Z and S mutations.[2] In the absence of these mutations, patients are sometimes

Table 10-4

Treatment Algorithm for Alpha-1-Antitrypsin

1. All patients with A1AT deficiency should be counseled with regard to elimination of possible sources of lung and liver injury

2. Patients with A1AT deficiency who are asymptomatic are not indicated to receive treatment but should be monitored for lung and liver disease

3. Patients with liver cirrhosis should be referred for liver transplantation

inappropriately diagnosed as having the "normal" MM genotype. In addition, genotyping will not detect null mutations because neither a Z nor S mutation is present; these patients would also be diagnosed with the MM genotype.

Previous reports have utilized liver biopsy and determination of the presence of periodic acid-Schiff–positive inclusions after diastase digestion (PAS-D) to diagnose A1AT deficiency.[1] Although liver biopsy is a valid and recommended procedure to assess liver disease severity in patients with A1AT deficiency, the prevalence of PAS-D inclusions is not 100% sensitive or specific for patients with the Z or S alleles. However, if PAS-D inclusions are seen during liver biopsy of a patient with chronic liver disease, the patient should be tested for A1AT deficiency.

Treatment

For individuals with A1AT who are asymptomatic, no treatment is indicated.[2] However, routine follow-up examinations for lung and liver disease are recommended.[2,3]

Augmentation therapy with exogenous infusion of purified pooled human plasma A1AT is beneficial in patients with A1AT-related lung disease, slowing the rate of decline of lung function, reducing mortality, and decreasing deterioration of lung tissue.[1] Unfortunately, augmentation therapy provides no benefit for patients with liver cirrhosis whose disease is the result of A1AT retention in hepatocytes as opposed to low circulating protein levels. For these patients, liver transplantation is indicated[1] and may be curative as liver replacement provides the recipient with the donor's A1AT phenotype.[2] All patients with A1AT deficiency should be counseled with regard to the elimination of possible sources of lung and liver injury (eg, smoking, alcohol abuse) that may worsen their condition, and hepatitis A and B vaccination may be recommended in patients with A1AT-related liver disease to prevent increased propensity for liver damage (Tables 10-4 and 10-5).[1]

Table 10-5

When to Refer Patients With Alpha-1-Antitrypsin

1. Patients with A1AT deficiency and COPD should be referred to a pulmonologist for disease monitoring once diagnosis is certain

2. Referral to a hepatologist is warranted for patients with A1AT deficiency and liver disease after initial diagnosis is established

COPD, chronic obstructive pulmonary disease.

WILSON'S DISEASE

Wilson's disease is an autosomal recessive disorder attributed to >300 different mutations in the copper dependent P-type ATPase, *ATP7B* gene located on human chromosome 13.[8] Wilson's disease occurs in approximately 1 in 30,000 to 1 in 100,000 individuals worldwide, with symptom onset between 20 to 30 years of age.[8] Mutations in the ATP7B gene prevent normal copper metabolism and excretion into bile. This enzyme transports copper to the Golgi apparatus for incorporation into ceruloplasmin, a major copper transporter in the blood, or to vesicles and vacuoles for excretion into the bile canaliculi. The resulting disruption of copper transport reduces the synthesis of ceruloplasmin and decreases the amount of copper excreted into bile. Also, copper accumulates within hepatocytes causing damage and eventually entering the bloodstream to be deposited in other organs, including the brain, kidneys, and corneas.

Clinical Pathophysiology

Wilson's disease manifests in a variety of clinical abnormalities, including neurologic and psychiatric dysfunction, ophthalmic abnormalities, and hepatic disease (Table 10-6).[8]

Approximately 40% to 50% of patients with Wilson's disease present with neurologic symptoms, including akinetic-rigid syndrome, pseudosclerosis, ataxia, and dystonic syndrome.[8] More subtle signs may also appear before onset of overt symptoms. Such signs comprise behavioral or mood changes, difficulty at school or work, deterioration of activities requiring hand-eye coordination (eg, handwriting), and cognitive deficits without overt hepatic encephalopathy. Neurologic manifestations occur most often in the third decade of life but may be present in children.[9] Children, however, are more

Table 10-6

Clinical Signs of Wilson's Disease

NEUROLOGIC/ PSYCHIATRIC MANIFESTATIONS	OPHTHALMIC MANIFESTATIONS	HEPATIC MANIFESTATIONS
Tremor	K-F rings	Persistently elevated serum ALT concentration
Choreiform movements	Brown or green pigmentation of the anterior and posterior lens (sunflower cataracts)	Chronic hepatitis
Parkinson-like akinetic-rigid syndrome		Cirrhosis (decompensated or compensated)
Gait disturbances	Night blindness	Fulminant hepatic failure with or without hemolytic anemia
Dysarthria	Exotropic strabismus	
Pseudobulbar palsy	Optic neuritis	
Rigid dystonia	Optic disc pallor	
Seizures		
Migraines		
Insomnia		
Depression		
Neuroses		
Personality changes		
Psychosis		

ALT, alanine aminotransferase; K-F, Kayser-Fleischer.
Adapted from Ala A, Walker AP, Ashkan K, Dooley JS, Schilsky ML. Wilson's disease. *Lancet.* 2007;369(9559):397-408. Copyright 2007, with permission from Elsevier.

likely to present with liver disease (eg, hepatic enlargement and abnormal serum alanine aminotransferase [ALT] levels) that are incidentally detected. Patients with symptomatic liver or neurologic symptoms may also display reduced serum uric acid concentrations associated with renal tubular dysfunction, although the diagnostic value of this parameter remains uncertain.

Fulminant hepatic failure is seen in 5% of patients with Wilson's disease (usually with Coombs-negative hemolytic anemia, renal failure, and increased copper concentrations in serum and urine).[8] Most of these patients, including children, have evidence of cirrhosis or massive liver necrosis and bridging fibrosis, low serum alkaline phosphatase concentrations, and all require urgent orthotopic liver transplantation. Patients may display compensated

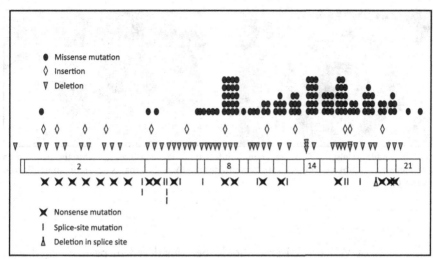

Figure 10-1. Identified genetic mutations in the Wilson's disease (ATP7B) gene.

cirrhosis or insidious cirrhosis with spider nevi, splenomegaly, portal hypertension, and ascites. Unfortunately, these symptoms are also typical of other forms of liver diseases (eg, chronic hepatitis).

Patients with Wilson's disease also display a clear ophthalmic manifestation known as Kayser-Fleischer (K-F) rings (Figure 10-2).[8]

These rings appear as brown discolorations around the outer margin of the cornea and are the result of copper deposition in the Descemet's membrane.[8] Similar rings may appear in patients with chronic liver diseases (eg, cholestasis and cryptogenic cirrhosis), however, and the presence of K-F rings alone should not be considered diagnostic of Wilson's disease.

Screening and Diagnosis

Screening

Family members of patients with Wilson's disease should be screened[9] because siblings of patients with Wilson's disease have a 25% chance of also having the disease based on its autosomal recessive hereditary pattern.[8] Such screening should include questions regarding a history of jaundice, liver disease, or neurologic dysfunction; a physical examination; serum copper and ceruloplasmin concentration testing; liver function tests; slit-lamp examination; and 24-hour urine copper concentration testing.[9] Molecular testing for specific ATP7B mutations should only be used if a specific mutation has been identified in an affected family member.

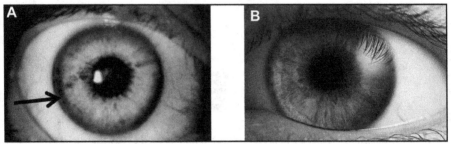

Figure 10-2. Kayser-Fleischer rings are a common feature of Wilson's disease.[8] Note the dark brown ring encircling the cornea of the eye with Wilson's disease (A, arrow) that is absent in an unaffected individual (B).

Diagnosis

Diagnosis of Wilson's disease should be considered in patients aged 3 to 55 years who have unexplained liver disease (Figure 10-3) and should be excluded in all patients with liver disease and neurologic or neuropsychiatric disturbances, hemolytic anemia, or low alkaline phosphatase.[9] In patients with neurologic symptoms, radiologic imaging (eg, magnetic resonance imaging, computed tomography) are warranted in addition to liver function testing to ascertain the potential presence of structural abnormalities in the basal ganglia.

Typically, ceruloplasmin levels are below normal (<20 mg/dL) in patients with Wilson's disease. Ceruloplasmin concentration results must be interpreted with care because concentrations are elevated by acute inflammation, pregnancy, estrogen supplementation, and use of oral contraceptive drugs. However, if low ceruloplasmin concentration and K-F rings are present and if urine copper concentration is also equivocal (ie, ≤100 μg copper/24 hours), diagnosis of Wilson's disease can be confirmed with a d-penicillamine challenge test, though this is rarely needed. This test is standardized in children and has been used in adults. In children, d-penicillamine 500 mg is administered twice during a 24-hour period (ie, an initial dose is followed by a second dose 12 hours later) and 24-hour urine copper concentration is measured. In individuals with a urine copper concentration >1600 μg/24 hours, a diagnosis of Wilson's disease can be definitively established.

Urine copper concentration is the established diagnostic test for Wilson's disease[9] with 24-hour copper levels >100 mg indicative of Wilson's disease. However, there is some debate among physicians as to the optimum copper concentration threshold for diagnosis of Wilson's disease since 16% to 23% of patients with Wilson's disease have copper concentrations <100 μg/24 hours. Because of this, the less-stringent concentration threshold of 40 μg/24 hours may be taken as indicative of Wilson's disease. Use of

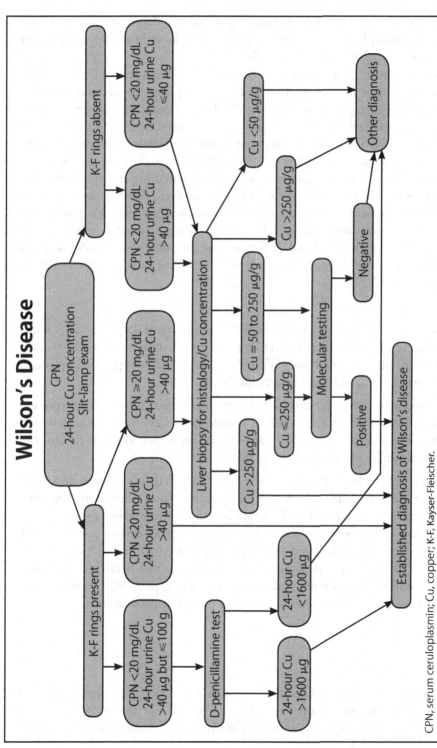

Figure 10-3. Algorithm for the diagnosis of Wilson's disease. All patients with unexplained liver disease should undergo diagnostic testing for Wilson's disease. (Modified with permission from Roberts EA, Schilsky ML; American Association for Study of Liver Diseases. Diagnosis and treatment of Wilson disease: an update. *Hepatology.* 2008;47(6):2089-2111.)

CPN, serum ceruloplasmin; Cu, copper; K-F, Kayser-Fleischer.

serum copper concentration has been suggested as a diagnostic parameter for Wilson's disease but it is difficult to evaluate the amount of copper bound or unbound to ceruloplasmin.

In some cases, liver biopsy and subsequent quantification of copper concentration may be necessary.[9] In liver biopsy samples, a copper concentration ≥250 µg/g dry weight is suggestive of Wilson's disease, but copper concentration may vary within the liver causing a potential misdiagnosis if a small area is biopsied. Thus, it is recommended that all biopsies to determine copper concentration are at least 1 to 2 cm. Common findings in patients with Wilson's disease include mild steatosis, glycogenated hepatocyte nuclei, and focal hepatocellular necrosis. Parenchymal damage, fibrosis, and cirrhosis may also be present. Mitochondrial and lysosome abnormalities may be visible upon ultrastructural analysis. Patients in whom diagnosis remains uncertain based on biochemical and clinical testing may undergo mutation analysis by whole-gene sequencing to firmly establish the diagnosis, though mutations are rarely found.

Special Populations

- *Autoimmune hepatitis.* Children with autoimmune hepatitis and adults with autoimmune hepatitis failing to respond to corticosteroid therapy should be evaluated for Wilson's disease.[9] However, distinguishing between the 2 disorders may be difficult.

- *Nonalcoholic fatty liver disease.* Patients with Wilson's disease often present with symptoms similar to that of nonalcoholic fatty liver disease but with less severe hepatic steatosis.[9] Patients may have both Wilson's disease and nonalcoholic fatty liver disease, though this is rare.

- *Acute liver failure.* Patients presenting with Wilson's disease and acute liver failure display prototypical characteristics, including Coombs-negative hemolytic anemia, coagulopathy unresponsive to vitamin K treatment, moderate increases in serum aminotransferases (<2000 IU/L), and normal-to-low serum alkaline phosphatase (<40 IU/L).[9] Rapid diagnosis of these patients is paramount because urgent liver transplantation is required and patients with acute liver failure associated with Wilson's disease receive the highest priority for liver transplantation.

Treatment

General population

Therapies for Wilson's disease encompass a variety of copper-chelating agents and promoters of copper excretion (Table 10-7).[9] These therapies must be maintained throughout the lifetime of the patient unless a liver transplantation is performed.

Table 10-7

Treatment Algorithm for Wilson's Disease

TREATMENT	RECOMMENDED DOSE	POTENTIAL SIDE EFFECTS	FOLLOW-UP PARAMETERS
D-penicillamine	Symptomatic: Adult: 1000 to 1500 mg/d Child: 20 mg/kg/d Asymptomatic: N/Eb Maintenance: 750 to 1000 mg/d	Fever Rash Proteinuria Lupus-like reaction Aplastic anemia Leukopenia Thrombocytopenia Nephrotic syndrome Degenerative changes in skin Hepatotoxicity	24-hour Cu excretion of 200 to 500 µg/dc Normalization of free serum Cu concentration
Trientine	Symptomatic: Adult: 750 to 1500 mg/d Child: 20 mg/kg/d Asymptomatic: N/R Maintenance: 750 or 1000 mg/d	Gastritis Anemia	24-hour Cu excretion of 200 to 500 µg/dc Normalization of free serum Cu concentration
Zinc	Symptomatic: N/R Asymptomatic: Adult: 150 mg/dd Child ≥50 kg: 150 mg/dd Child <50 kg: 75 mg/dd Maintenance: 150 mg/dd	Gastritis Zinc accumulation Changes in immune function	24-hour Cu excretion of <75 µg/d Normalization of free serum Cu concentration Urine zinc concentration to measure compliance
Tetrathio-molybdate	Experimental therapy in US; not commercially available	Bone marrow suppression Hepatotoxicity Neurologic dysfunction	N/A

Cu, copper; N/A, not applicable; N/E, not established; N/R, not recommended; (a) therapy should begin at 250 to 500 mg/d and be increased by 250 mg every 4 to 7 days until maximum dose is reached to improve tolerability; (b) dose of ≥1 g/d combined with a low-copper diet demonstrated efficacy in a trial of 53 asymptomatic patients;[10] (c) concentration <200 µg/d may indicate nonadherence or overtreatment; (d) measured as elemental zinc.

The first drug used for treatment of Wilson's disease was d-penicillamine in 1956.[9] This cysteine derivative promotes the urinary excretion of copper and is a general metal chelator. Numerous studies have reported the beneficial effect of d-penicillamine for patients with Wilson's disease, but side effects including initial worsening of neurologic symptoms are common. Severe side effects requiring drug discontinuation in approximately 30% of patients typically occur within the first 3 weeks of treatment and include fever, cutaneous eruptions, lymphadenopathy, neutropenia, and proteinuria. Development of other side effects (eg, nephrotoxicity, lupus-like syndrome, bone marrow toxicity, and hepatotoxicity) may also occur. Because of these potential effects, d-penicillamine is no longer recommended as first-line therapy.[8,9]

Trientine was developed for treatment of patients who were intolerant of d-penicillamine and is now considered first-line therapy because of its low incidence of side effects.[8,9] Trientine promotes copper excretion by the kidneys and may mobilize different copper stores than those affected by d-penicillamine.[8,9] Neurologic worsening at the beginning of trientine therapy has been reported but is less frequent than with d-penicillamine. The typical adult dose of trientine is 750 to 1500 mg/d and should be given until copper excretion concentrations normalize. Thereafter, patients should be maintained on trientine alone or in combination with zinc but at a lower dose (750 or 1000 mg/d).

Zinc was first used for Wilson's disease in the 1960s.[8,9] It interferes with uptake of dietary copper in the gastrointestinal tract by inducing expression of the metal chelator protein metallothionein in enterocytes. Once bound to metallothionein, copper is excreted into the feces. Zinc has been shown to be an effective treatment for asymptomatic patients and is typically used as maintenance therapy given 3 times a day. The 3 times daily dosing may deter compliance, but zinc must be taken at least twice daily to be effective. In addition, poor tolerability of zinc has been reported but this is generally a reaction to the salt with which zinc is compounded (eg, acetate) and may improve upon use of a different ionic compound.

Ammonium tetrathiomolybdate is an experimental chelating agent that is being examined for treatment of Wilson's disease.[8,9] Results from a phase 3 trial of tetrathiomolybdate and zinc combination therapy in patients with Wilson's disease and neurologic dysfunction recovered 81% of their neurologic function after 8 weeks of tetrathiomolybdate and 3 years of zinc maintenance therapy.[11] However, further clinical trials are necessary to establish the efficacy and tolerability of tetrathiomolybdate (Tables 10-8 and 10-9).

Special Populations

- *Decompensated cirrhosis.* Patients with decompensated cirrhosis without hepatic encephalopathy should receive either d-penicillamine

Table 10-8

Treatment Algorithm for Wilson's Disease

1. Asymptomatic patients may receive zinc 150 mg/day to prevent elevation of copper concentration

2. Symptomatic patients should receive trientine 750 to 1500 mg/day until normalization of copper excretion

3. Patients who experience normalization of copper excretion during initial trientine therapy should be continually maintained on lower doses (750 or 1000 mg/day) of trientine

4. Maintenance therapy must continue throughout the lifetime of the patient unless a liver transplantation is performed

Table 10-9

When to Refer Patients With Wilson's Disease for Liver Transplantation

1. Patients with acute liver failure should be referred for transplantation and closely monitored until the procedure can be performed

2. Patients with decompensated cirrhosis who do not respond to treatment with d-penicillamine or trientine in combination with zinc should be referred for transplantation immediately

(25 mg/kg for children) or trientine (500 mg in adults; 10 mg/kg in children) in combination with zinc (50 mg for adults; 25 mg for children).[9,12] In such cases, administration of the chelater and zinc therapy must be separated by at least 5 hours to prevent chelation of the zinc in the gut.[9,12] Patients who respond to this regimen may be transitioned onto zinc or trientine monotherapy after 3 to 6 months.

- *Pregnancy.* Treatment should be maintained during pregnancy to prevent acute liver failure, but the dose of chelating agent (eg, d-penicillamine or trientine) should be reduced by 25% to 50%.[9] If zinc is used, dose adjustments are not necessary. Women who receive d-penicillamine should not breastfeed. Rare instances of birth defects in patients who received treatment for Wilson's disease during pregnancy have been reported, but the contribution of d-penicillamine or trientine to these defects are unknown.

Table 10-10

Disorders Associated With Hemochromatosis

ACQUIRED	HEREDITARY
Dietary	Genetic hemochromatosis
Parenteral	• HFE
Inflammation-associated anemia	• TfR2
Transfusion-dependent iron-loading anemias	• HAMP
Long-term hemodialysis	• FPN
Chronic liver disease	FPN disease
Alloimmune neonatal hemochroma-tosis[a]	Aceruloplasminemia
	Atransferrinemia
African hemochromatosis[b]	DMT1 deficiency
	Hereditary iron-loading anemi-as[c]
	H ferritin mutation
	Friedreich's ataxia
	Porphyria cutanea tarda

DMT1, divalent metal transporter 1; FPN, ferroportin; HAMP, hepcidin; HFE, human hemochromatosis protein; HJV, hemojuvelin; TfR2, transferrin receptor 2. (a) Once considered hereditary, it is now believed to be caused by maternal alloimmunity to the fetal liver. (b) Particularly frequent among Africans in sub-Saharan regions who drink a traditional beer brewed in nongalvanized steel drums. (c) Parenchymal iron overload is detectable before transfusion. It is caused by inefficient erythropoiesis and HAMP downregulation.

Reproduced from Pietrangelo A. Hereditary hemochromatosis: pathogenesis, diagnosis, and treatment. *Gastroenterology.* 2010;139(2):393-408. Copyright 2010, with permission from Elsevier.

HEREDITARY HEMOCHROMATOSIS

Hemochromatosis is a disorder of iron metabolism and excretion resulting in the toxic accumulation of iron in parenchymal cells of vital organs.[13] The most predominant form of iron overload is caused by genetic mutations within iron regulatory genes (ie, hereditary hemochromatosis, Table 10-10).[13] These disorders need to be distinguished from other chronic liver disorders (eg, alcoholic or nonalcoholic fatty liver or viral liver disease) that may cause elevation of systemic iron levels particularly serum ferritin.[14]

The pathophysiology and pathology of HH is complex and variable depending on the interaction of multiple genetic and environmental factors.[13]

Various gene polymorphisms only predispose individuals to hemochromatosis; additional genetic or environmental factors are required for development of the disease leading to a variable penetrance. The most common genetic variant associated with HH is a polymorphism (C282Y) in the gene encoding human hemochromatosis protein (HFE), a protein that sensitizes hepatocytes to low levels of iron. Prevalence of this genetic alteration varies by ethnic group, with approximately 0.4% of white individuals being homozygous for the mutation and 9.6% being heterozygous.[15] In contrast, 0.014% of African Americans, 0.027% of Mexican Americans, and 0% of Asians are homozygous C282Y individuals. However, only 38% to 50% of patients homozygous for C282Y polymorphism develop HH.[13] Additional polymorphisms of the HFE gene (eg, H63D) have also been described in the general population but are rarely associated with disease. Other genetic abnormalities, including polymorphisms in genes for ferroportin (FPN), hepcidin (HAMP), hemojuvelin (HJV), and transferrin receptor 2 (TfR2), have also been associated with HH but are generally less prevalent than the C282Y HFE variation. Any mutation within genes responsible for normal iron homeostasis, however, may contribute to HH.

Iron Homeostasis

Dietary iron is absorbed from the small intestines by divalent metal transporter 1 (DMT1) within enterocytes.[13,15] Iron may then be stored by the enterocytes or released into the bloodstream depending on physiological need that is sensed by ferroportin (FPN). Ferroportin binds HAMP, which is released by the liver in response to excess iron. When HAMP is bound to FPN, the iron transporter is internalized and degraded; however, when HAMP levels fall indicating low body-iron levels, FPN transports intracellular iron into the bloodstream.[13] In addition, hepatocytes sense blood iron concentrations via signaling induced by transferrin binding to TFR1 receptors and subsequent intracellular signaling involving proteins such as HJV and TFR2. Disruption of any of these signaling pathways whether via genetic mutation or environmental and metabolic factors (eg, alcohol consumption, obesity)[14] may result in excess iron via inappropriate release and storage of intracellular iron.[13] Interestingly, dietary iron is not the predominant cause of increased iron concentration in HH. Rather, increased release of iron by macrophages during the process of red blood cell destruction appears to be the main contributor.[13] The molecular signals underlying this mechanism remain unknown.

Clinical Pathophysiology

The presentation of HH is variable both in time of onset and characteristics and depends on the genetic polymorphisms underlying the disease (Table 10-11).[13]

Table 10-11

Characteristics of Various Forms of Hemochromatosis

HEMO-CHRO-MATOSIS	AGE OF ONSET (YEARS)	ETHNIC POPULA-TION	GENDER	CLINICAL PARA-METERS	COMMON SYMPTOMS
HFE	40 to 50	White	Male	Elevated SF concentra-tion Increased TS	Fatigue Dark skin Arthralgia Hepato-megaly
TfR2	30 to 40	White or nonwhite	Male or female	Elevated SF concentra-tion Increased TS	Cardio-myopathy Endocrino-pathy Liver disease
HJV or HAMP	15 to 20	White or nonwhite	Male or female	High SF con-centration High TS	Impotence Amenorrhea Cardio-myopathy
FPN	10 to 80	White or nonwhite	Male or female	Unexplained increase of SF concen-tration Normal TS	Hyper-ferritinemia

FPN, ferroportin; HAMP, hepcidin; HFE, human hemochromatosis protein; HJV, hemojuvelin; SF, serum ferritin; TfR2, transferrin receptor 2; TS, transferrin saturation

Adapted from Pietrangelo A. Hereditary hemochromatosis: pathogenesis, diagnosis, and treatment. *Gastroenterology*. 2010;139(2):393-408. Copyright 2010, with permission from Elsevier.

In the past, the most common symptoms of HH were unexplained cirrhosis, bronze-colored skin, diabetes, joint inflammation, and heart disease. However, increased screening and awareness have allowed the disease to be detected earlier. Thus, the most common presenting symptoms now are fatigue, malaise, arthralgia, and hepatomegaly and many patients are discovered through routine laboratory testing with no symptoms. Most patients (24% to 32%) have elevated liver enzyme concentrations[13] and patients with cirrhosis are at increased risk for the development of HCC.

Cirrhosis occurs in 4.4% to 11.8% of male patients homozygous for the C282Y polymorphism and is observed in females much less frequently (up to 2.7% of patients). Increased risk of cirrhosis has been associated with age, increased serum ferritin levels,[18-20] and mutations in inflammatory[19] and oxidative stress–related genes.[20] In addition, patients with excess intake of alcohol may develop earlier and more severe liver fibrosis compared with patients who abstain from alcohol, and patients with nonalcoholic fatty liver disease have an increased risk of fibrosis.[14] Generally, mild liver fibrosis is reversible with treatment, but hemochromatosis-related morbidity occurs in 10% to 33% of patients.[13] However, early diagnosis and therapeutic intervention of hemochromatosis may reduce the risk of secondary complications (eg, type 2 diabetes) and enhance the overall survival of patients.

Screening and Diagnosis

Screening

Screening of individuals who are related to patients with HH is possible with genetic testing, but the risks and benefits should be thoroughly discussed with the individual.[21] Given the variety of genetic mutations potentially involved in a negative test for HFE may give the individual a false sense of security. In addition, the cost and social issues involved in genetic testing, including the social impact of disease labeling and insurability, should be understood before testing. Therefore, in most cases, genetic testing should be restricted to family members of those with a known mutation and with liver disease and high transferrin saturation and ferritin.

Diagnosis

Other liver disorders, such as nonalcoholic fatty liver disease, may also result in elevated iron levels and should be excluded before genetic testing for hereditary hemochromatosis is performed.[14] For patients with a family history and all patients with abnormal LFTs, transferrin saturation and serum ferritin concentration should be evaluated. Patients with abnormal levels should have additional procedures performed as outlined in Figure 10-4.[13,15] In general, transferrin saturation >45% and serum ferritin levels >200 µg/L for women or >300 µg/L for men are suggestive of HH.[21]

Patients with a high transferrin saturation but normal ferritin concentration indicates that alternative diagnoses should be sought. In patients with normal TS and high ferritin concentration, other causes of high ferritin (eg, inflammation) should be excluded. If symptoms persist, liver biopsy or MRI to examine the concentration and pattern of iron accumulation should be performed. Presence of iron overload in these cases may indicate non-HFE (usually ferroportion hemochromatosis). White patients with high TS

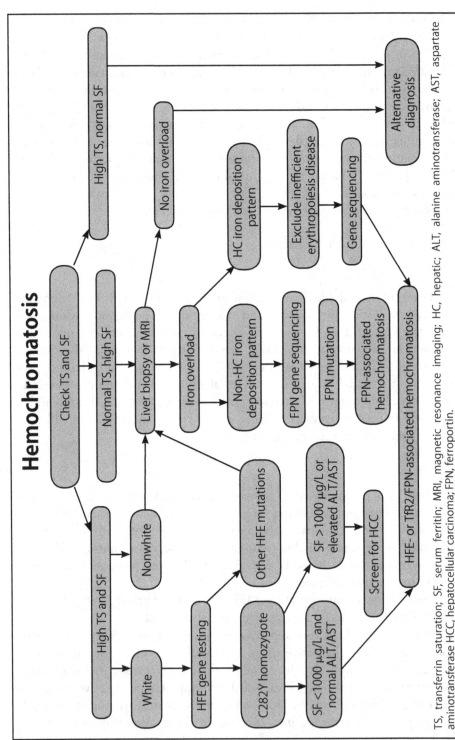

Figure 10-4. Algorithm for the work-up and diagnosis of hemochromatosis.

TS, transferrin saturation; SF, serum ferritin; MRI, magnetic resonance imaging; HC, hepatic; ALT, alanine aminotransferase; AST, aspartate aminotransferase HCC, hepatocellular carcinoma; FPN, ferroportin.

and elevated ferritin levels should be tested for mutation in the HFE gene. If patients are homozygous for the C282Y polymorphism, a diagnosis of HFE-related hemochromatosis can be established. If other mutations are observed in the HFE gene, other comorbidities should be ruled out and a liver biopsy performed to determine the degree and pattern of iron accumulation. Heterogeneous distribution of iron suggests hematological disorders with inefficient erythropoiesis; therefore, these disorders should be ruled out before additional testing. If other hematologic disorders are not present, diagnosis of HFE- or TfR2-associated hemochromatosis may be concluded with gene sequencing.

Treatment

After diagnosis of HH, referral to a hepatologist or hematologist is recommended.[15] This is because the primary treatment for HH is therapeutic phlebotomy, which requires careful monitoring. No standard recommendations for the initiation and conduct of phlebotomy in HH have been developed, making clinical expertise with phlebotomy essential. Phlebotomy is usually initiated when serum ferritin levels are above normal (ie, >200 μg/L for women or >300 μg/L for men) with the goal of creating an iron-depleted status in the patient.[13,15] Approximately one unit (400 to 500 mL) of blood should be removed weekly for 1 to 2 years monitoring hemoglobin and ferritin levels frequently.[13] In elderly patients or patients with comorbidities, removal of 0.5 units of blood is standard because these populations are less tolerant of an anemic state.[15] After 1 to 2 years, removal of 1 to 2 units for women or 3 to 4 units for men per year is usually sufficient to keep serum ferritin levels between 50 and 100 μg/L.[13,15] Ferritin levels should be measured regularly, and yearly examination of transferrin saturation is necessary.[15] Patients who are intolerant of phlebotomy due to hematologic disorders associated with ineffective erythropoiesis or hemolysis may receive subcutaneous therapy with the chelating agent deferoxamine at 2 g/day over 8 hours; however, the efficacy of deferoxamine has not been well established (Tables 10-12 and 10-13).

REFERENCES

1. American Thoracic Society/European Respiratory Society statement: standards for the diagnosis and management of individuals with alpha-1 antitrypsin deficiency. *Am J Respir Crit Care Med.* 2003;168(7):818-900.

2. Sandhaus RA. Alpha-1 antitrypsin deficiency: whom to test, whom to treat? *Semin Respir Crit Care Med.* 2010;31(3):343-347.

3. Silverman EK, Sandhaus RA. Clinical practice. Alpha1-antitrypsin deficiency. *N Engl J Med.* 2009;360(26):2749-2757.

Table 10-12

Diagnostic/Treatment Algorithm for Hemochromatosis

1. Indiscriminate genetic testing is not recommended in the United States[21]

2. Patients with persistent ferritin >1000 µg/L should be evaluated for other causes of hyperferritinemia[13]

3. Phlebotomy should be performed weekly for 1 to 2 years[13,15]

4. Once a consistent iron-deficient status is achieved, phlebotomy is necessary only once or twice a year[13,15]

Table 10-13

When to Refer Patients With Hemochromatosis for Specialty Care

1. Patients requiring intensive genetic testing for HH diagnosis should be referred

2. Patients should be referred to a hematologist or hepatologist after diagnosis of HH

HH, hereditary hemochromatosis.

4. Lomas DA, Mahadeva R. α1-antitrypsin polymerization and the serpinopathies: pathobiology and prospects for therapy. *J Clin Invest.* 2002;110(11):1585-1590.

5. Lawless MW, Greene CM, Mulgrew A, Taggart CC, O'Neill SJ, McElvaney NG. Activation of endoplasmic reticulum-specific stress responses associated with the conformational disease Z alpha 1-antitrypsin deficiency. *J Immunol.* 2004;172(9):5722-5726.

6. Petrache I, Hajjar J, Campos M. Safety and efficacy of alpha-1-antitrypsin augmentation therapy in the treatment of patients with alpha-1-antitrypsin deficiency. *Biologics.* 2009;3:193-204.

7. Hogarth DK, Rachelefsky G. Screening and familial testing of patients for α1-antitrypsin deficiency. *Chest.* 2008;133(4):981-988.

8. Ala A, Walker AP, Ashkan K, Dooley JS, Schilsky ML. Wilson's disease. *Lancet.* 2007;369(9559):397-408.

9. Roberts EA, Schilsky ML. Diagnosis and treatment of Wilson disease: an update. *Hepatology.* 2008;47(6):2089-2111.

10. Sternlieb I, Scheinberg IH. Prevention of Wilson's disease in asymptomatic patients. *N Engl J Med.* 1968;278(7):352-359.

11. Brewer GJ, Askari F, Lorincz MT, et al. Treatment of Wilson disease with ammonium tetrathiomolybdate: IV. Comparison of tetrathiomolybdate and trientine in a double-blind study of treatment of the neurologic presentation of Wilson disease. *Arch Neurol.* 2006;63(4):521-527.

12. Santos Silva EE, Sarles J, Buts JP, Sokal EM. Successful medical treatment of severely decompensated Wilson disease. *J Pediatr.* 1996;128(2):285-287.

13. Pietrangelo A. Hereditary hemochromatosis: pathogenesis, diagnosis, and treatment. *Gastroenterology.* 2010;139(2):393-408.

14. Deugnier Y, Brissot P, Loréal O. Iron and the liver: update 2008. *J Hepatol.* 2008;48(suppl 1):S113-S123.

15. Yen AW, Fancher TL, Bowlus CL. Revisiting hereditary hemochromatosis: current concepts and progress. *Am J Med.* 2006;119(5):391-399.

16. Aigner E, Theurl I, Theurl M, et al. Pathways underlying iron accumulation in human nonalcoholic fatty liver disease. *Am J Clin Nutr.* 2008;87(5):1374-1383.

17. Mitsuyoshi H, Yasui K, Harano Y, et al. Analysis of hepatic genes involved in the metabolism of fatty acids and iron in nonalcoholic fatty liver disease. *Hepatol Res.* 2009;39(4):366-373.

18. Morrison ED, Brandhagen DJ, Phatak PD, et al. Serum ferritin level predicts advanced hepatic fibrosis among US patients with phenotypic hemochromatosis. *Ann Intern Med.* 2003;138(8):627-633.

19. Osterreicher CH, Datz C, Stickel F, et al. TGF-beta1 codon 25 gene polymorphism is associated with cirrhosis in patients with hereditary hemochromatosis. *Cytokine.* 2005;31(2):142-148.

20. Osterreicher CH, Datz C, Stickel F, et al. Association of myeloperoxidase promotor polymorphism with cirrhosis in patients with hereditary hemochromatosis. *J Hepatol.* 2005;42(6):914-919.

21. Qaseem A, Aronson M, Fitterman N, Snow V, Weiss KB, Owens DK, for the Clinical Efficacy Assessment Subcommittee of the American College of Physicians. Screening for hereditary hemochromatosis: a clinical practice guideline from the American College of Physicians. *Ann Intern Med.* 2005;143(7):517-521.

Financial
Disclosures

Dr. George G. Abdelsayed has no financial or proprietary interest in the materials presented herein.

Dr. Patrick Basu has no financial or proprietary interest in the materials presented herein.

Dr. Robert S. Brown Jr receives grant and research support from Vertex, Janssen, Gilead, and Merck. He is a consultant for Gilead and Vertex and is on the speaker's bureau for Vertex, Gilead, Merck, and Genentech. Columbia University receives research support from Gilead, Merck, Vertex, Janssen, and Boehringer.

Dr. Blaire E. Burman has no financial or proprietary interest in the materials presented herein.

Dr. Sanjiv Chopra has not disclosed any relevant financial relationships.

Dr. Michael Einstein has no financial or proprietary interest in the materials presented herein.

Dr. Scott A. Fink has not disclosed any relevant financial relationships.

Dr. Mark W. Russo has not disclosed any relevant financial relationships.

Dr. Niraj James Shah has no financial or proprietary interest in the materials presented herein.

Dr. Eva Urtasun Sotil is a consultant and speaker for Otsuka Pharmaceuticals and a consultant for Salix Pharmaceuticals.

Dr. James F. Trotter is a consultant for Novartis.

Dr. Elizabeth C. Verna has no financial or proprietary interest in the materials presented herein.

Index

Printed in the United States
by Baker & Taylor Publisher Services